What People Are Saying about Discover Wellness

"Wellness causes prosperity, and to benefit and profit you need to read, absorb, and use the great wisdom in Discover Wellness. Lifelong wellness is our individual and collective quest to save our economy. Drs. Hoffman and Deitch are brilliant geniuses and leading-edge thinkers, as well as friends of mine, with solutions to a wiser, healthier, and richer future for you and your family."

> - Mark Victor Hansen
>   Co-author of the International Bestselling Series
>   *Chicken Soup for the Soul*

"This is the most important subject that anyone can read and learn about at this time. This sensational book covers it all...beautifully done and wonderfully written...enjoy!"

> - Michael Gerber
>   Bestselling Author of *The E-Myth*

"Informative, insightful, and inspirational...this book is a treasure trove of useful, pragmatic, down-to-earth material that each and every reader could begin to put to work in his or her life immediately—the fact that it is also a pleasant and easy read only adds to its value. Congratulations."

> - Dr. Gerard W. Clum, D.C.
>   President, Life Chiropractic College West
>   President, World Federation of Chiropractic

"Discover Wellness, How Staying Healthy Can Make You Rich shines a revealing light on our current health care system and offers us a compelling path to healing our individual and collective body, mind, and soul."

> - Dr. David Simon, M.D.
>   Medical Director,
>   The Chopra Center for Wellbeing

"Dr. Bob Hoffman and Dr. Jason A. Deitch are visionary leaders in the field of human performance and wellness. Their brilliant new book, Discover Wellness, How Staying Healthy Can Make You Rich, offers a clear roadmap to lead you out of America's current health care crisis and into a state of extraordinary health, well-being, and abundance every day of your life."

- Debbie Ford
  Bestselling Author of *The Best Year of Your Life*

"The Wellness Revolution is indeed here and the wisdom from Discover Wellness, How Staying Healthy Can Make You Rich is the blueprint for any fitness and wellness professional interested in bringing greater prosperity and success into their practice."

- Peter Davis
  Co-founder, IDEA Health & Fitness Association, and InnerIDEA
  World's largest association for health and fitness professionals

"Leonardo da Vinci wrote 'Learn to preserve your own health.' In this wise and wonderful book, Dr. Bob Hoffman and Dr. Jason A. Deitch show us how to follow the Maestro's advice in the modern world."

- Michael J. Gelb
  Author of *How to Think Like Leonardo da Vinci* and
  Body Learning: An Introduction to the Alexander Technique

"Wellness is without doubt the model needed to shift out of our reliance and dependency of the fatally flawed conventional medical system, and this book will help you start in that direction."

- Dr. Joe Mercola, D.O.
  Founder of Mercola.com
  The world's most visited natural health Web site

"As a family physician and concerned citizen, I encourage you to take an active role in your own health, and I have hopes that America's health care system is able to rediscover that you, your family, and your community are where health care happens. I encourage you to Discover Wellness. Please enjoy this powerful and important book."

- Dr. Michael Zimmerman, M.D.

"In my 25 years of providing financial planning services to high net worth individuals, celebrities, executives and business owners, I've discovered the most overlooked aspect of building wealth is building health so you can enjoy the fruits of your labor. The strategies in Discover Wellness, How Staying Healthy Can Make You Rich focus on providing effective solutions for you to reduce your risk of losing not only your money, but your most important asset, your health. This is a perfect tool for all financial advisors seeking to provide clients an effective solution to building true wealth."

- Paul Auslander, CFP
  CEO, American Financial Advisors

"The cost of our employees' health care has a direct effect on our profitability. The wisdom in Discover Wellness, How Staying Healthy Can Make You Rich is not only a message of better health: it will help our company increase profits for years to come. We've been desperately seeking solutions to the skyrocketing costs of our employees' health care; this book offers great insight into how to provide win/win solutions for us and our employees. THANK YOU!"

- Steve Allen
  CEO, Silicon Valley Staffing Group

"Thank you for creating a terrific book that helps more people appreciate the wellness lifestyle."

- Kevin MacDonald
  Director, The Claremont Resort and Spa, Berkeley, California

"Discover Wellness gives you a glimpse of a life of never getting old."

-Dr. Dick Versendaal, D.C.

"To discover wellness, one needs only to discover one's self. The balance of illness or wellness, prosperity or lack, is held quite simply in one's awareness of one's own capacity. Discover Wellness provides the tools necessary to bring forth that awareness with great certainty for anyone interested. And we all are. Thank you Dr. Bob and Dr. Jason for your energies of healing and wholeness for humankind! I will share this most informative tool with my audiences globally."

- Dr. Sue Morter, D.C.
  DynamicLifeTraining.com

"Our company has been on the front lines of the Wellness Revolution for over ten years providing wellness programs and wellness coaching to large corporations and small businesses across America. Discover Wellness, How Staying Healthy Can Make You Rich reveals just how incredibly expensive our current sick-care model of health care really is, and provides practical and effective solutions for both employers and employees to work together and profit together. This book is a must-have for any employer seeking to reduce health care costs and inspire their employees to be healthier, more productive, and more effective at what they do."

- Arlene K. Singer,
  CEO, WellCall, Inc.

"Wellness is simultaneously the most important and most confusing topic for the average consumer. One's life depends on it, but there is so much incoherent noise about wellness that many give up trying to discover it. Discover Wellness is a literal lifeline that clarifies the path and gives one direction on living the wellness lifestyle. Read it for a better life."

- Dr. Patrick Gentempo, Jr., D.C.
CEO, Creating Wellness Alliance, Inc.

Discover Wellness
How Staying Healthy Can Make You Rich

Dr. Bob Hoffman, D.C. • Dr. Jason A. Deitch, D.C.

616
Hof

Legalese

Due to the present state of our country, we find it unfortunate but necessary to include the following statements regarding liability. The information contained in this book is based upon the research and personal and professional experiences of the authors. It is not intended as a substitute for consulting with your physician or other health care providers. Any attempt to diagnose and treat an illness should be done under the direction of a health care professional.

The publisher and authors do not advocate the use of any particular health care protocol, but believe the information in this book should be available to the public. The publisher and authors are not responsible for any adverse effects or consequences resulting from the use of the suggestions, procedures, products, and services discussed in this book. Should the reader have any questions concerning the appropriateness of any procedures or products mentioned, the authors and publisher strongly suggest consulting a professional health care advisor.

If you cannot agree to the above, then please close this book and do not read any further. Your continued reading is your acknowledgment and agreement to hold harmless everyone connected with the production of this book.

One more thing before we get started, this book was written by two primary authors with the help of a team of health care professionals, researchers, and writers. We have chosen to write this book in the first person for the sake of convenience and readability.

Center Path Publishing
3459 Washington Drive
Suite 202
Eagan, MN 55122

Cover design by Kerry Martyr

Library of Congress Cataloging-in-Publication Data

Hoffman, Bob.
  Discover wellness : how staying healthy can make you rich / by Bob Hoffman and Jason Deitch. -- [2nd ed.]
    p. cm.
  First ed. published in 2006, entered under: Deitch, Jason.
  Includes bibliographical references.
  ISBN 978-1-933889-27-6 (alk. paper)
  1. Health--Miscellanea. 2. Medical care--Miscellanea. 3. Social medicine--Miscellanea. I. Deitch, Jason. Discover wellness. II. Title.

RA776D45 2007
616--dc22

                          2006100726

4/07
BOT

Table of Contents

Dedication

We dedicate this book to you,
the person who has the power to make the choice
to shift from what is toward what can be…

Acknowledgments

A book project such as this cannot be done alone. We thank everyone along the way who has helped teach us, support us, love us, and inspire us to put forth the effort to complete this most exciting project. First and most importantly, we would like to thank our wives Sharon Hoffman and Melanie Deitch for their years of love and support while we have embarked on our mission of service and dedication to making a positive difference in the world.

We also want to say thank you to our children Tara, Amanda, Chelsey, Coby, and Noah for being our inspiration of hope and our experience of love that transcends words and provides the source of our deeper purpose of working towards a future world of wellness. We say thank you to our parents for their years of love and care and always believing that we can do "whatever your heart desires." We believed you.

We thank all of the people at The Masters Circle with whom we have the privilege of getting to work everyday and who help make our dreams a reality.

In addition, we could not be more grateful to those people who have given us their hearts and shown us their passion in helping us make this book a reality. We thank our publisher Dr. Todd Berntson at Center Path Publishing and his great team.

Lastly, we would like to thank the people who have inspired us over the years. Dr. D.D. Palmer, Dr. B.J. Palmer, Dr. Sid Williams, Dr. Gerry Clum, Dr. Bill Remling, Dr. Larry Markson, Dr. Dennis Perman, Dr. Patrick Gentempo, Dr. Arno Burnier, Dr. Sue Morter, Dr. Dick Versendaal, Dr. Tedd Koren, Dr. Scott Donkin, Dr. Jeff Spencer, Dr. Joe Mercola, Mark Victor Hansen, Robin Sharma, Michael Gerber, Michael Gelb, Peter Davis, Dr. Michael Zimmerman, Dr. David Simon, Dr. Deepak Chopra, and Anthony Robbins. We thank you!

Foreword
by Robin Sharma

Ultimately, our lives are shaped by our conversations, and I hope that this wonderful book is one of those conversations that will shape your life. Years ago, as you may have read in my book *The Monk Who Sold His Ferrari*, I left my previous life of being a successful lawyer for a life of purpose and authenticity. Not to say that you can't have purpose, authenticity and a Ferrari—it's just that I didn't. Nothing is wrong with making money—it's just that I placed it above meaning.

Since then, I have made it a habit and a lifestyle to take risks and follow my dreams. I now spend my professional life traveling the planet to help people and organizations become extraordinary.

What I have learned over the years as an executive coach working with billionaires, CEOs, celebrity entrepreneurs, and speaking to thousands of organizations is that a lot of people sacrifice health for wealth. They take their health for granted until they lose it. That's why this book is so valuable.

Dr. Bob Hoffman's and Dr. Jason A. Deitch's message of making your life a priority by putting your health at the top of your list is critical if you want to create a world-class life for yourself and your family. True, creating a remarkable life requires discipline and hard work. But I've learned that the best things in life offer the greatest challenges and require the greatest sacrifice.

Norman Cousins once said, "The great tragedy is not death, it's what we allow to die inside of us while we live." When you are on your deathbed, you're not thinking about how much money you have or how much you have accomplished. The questions people generally ask on their deathbeds are:

1. *Have I lived wisely?*
2. *Have I loved well?*
3. *Have I served greatly?*

I often reflect on what prevents people from having the discipline to do the inner work necessary to focus on promoting their own health and wellness. I have found that there are four primary factors that keep us from making changes we ideally would want to make.

Fear: We fear leaving the safe harbor of the known for the unknown. The key is to manage the fear by doing the very thing that frightens you. Do it until you are no longer scared.

Failure: Since we don't want to fail, we don't try. That keeps us from taking the first step to improve our health, or deepen our workplace relationships, or try to realize some career or personal dream. In my mind, the only failure in life is the failure to try. I deeply believe that the greatest risk you can ever take is in not taking risks.

Forgetting: We are ready to change the world after imbibing some inspirational wisdom, but as soon as everyday life intrudes again, we are diverted from that goal and it slips from our mind. Instead, keep your commitments in focus. Write them on three-by-five-inch cards and place them on your bathroom mirror if you have to.

(Lack of) ***Faith:*** Too many people are cynical, convinced personal development suggestions don't work. That stems from a time when they were filled with possibilities and hope, perhaps as a kid, and failed at something. Instead, you need to view failure and risk as the highway to success.

If your fear of the unknown is what stops you from adopting a wellness lifestyle, then I advise you to be fearless, to run towards the problem rather than run away from it. The greatest risk in life is not taking risks. As I write in my book *The Greatness Guide*, on our deathbeds we never regret the risks we took, only the opportunities we didn't seize.

If fear of failure is what stops you from creating the life of your dreams, then I recommend you take little steps towards your goal over 30 days so it can become a habit. Improve one percent each day. Over time you'll get to a place you never imagined.

If you are forgetting to make healthy choices, how about putting a photo of your ideal body on the bathroom mirror to remind yourself of what you visualize yourself to look like?

If you don't have the faith to think you can do it, then I wonder, what bill of goods have you sold yourself as to what's possible? What false assumptions are you making in terms of what you cannot have, do, and be? Your thinking creates your reality. Your thoughts form your world.

It is my true passion to help people create the world-class lifestyle of their dreams. *Discover Wellness, How Staying Healthy Can Make You Rich* is a great tool to help you do just that. By first realizing the consequences of our present actions, we get an emotional understanding of both the physical and financial impact that the most common lifestyle-related health conditions have on our lives.

Dr. Bob and Dr. Jason provide a step-by-step guide to understanding what to do to make healthy choices part of our lifestyle. They show us not only what the costs are but also how we can profit in every way. This is a guide to creating a life of health and wealth that will give us valuable new insight and perspective into how wellness will impact our global economy in the future.

I urge you to use *Discover Wellness* as a handbook to reach your greatness personally, to enrich your life emotionally, reach more of your potential professionally, improve your profits financially, and most importantly, to make a greater contribution socially.

May this book help you create an extraordinary life about which you can be proud.

- Robin Sharma
  Bestselling author of *The Monk Who Sold His Ferrari* and *The Greatness Guide*

I

Introduction: America's Health Care Crisis

A perfect storm has been brewing just over the horizon and is heading this way, bringing with it a torrent that has the power to ruin the lives of all those it touches. The leaders of our nation have seen the forecasts and are wringing their hands not knowing what to do about it. This storm will wreak more havoc than any natural disaster in history, leaving millions of Americans sick and unprotected—at least the lucky ones. The unlucky ones will not survive.

The name of this storm is not a common name like Katrina, Andrew, or Wilma. It is called "America's Health Care Crisis." Most people are completely unaware of how big this storm is, but as with other disastrous events in our history, the day will soon come when the world as we all know it will end. Early signs of the looming storm have already begun to reach us. Just consider these facts:

- *Every 30 seconds in the United States someone files for bankruptcy due to a serious health problem.[1] According to a recent study by Harvard University, 50 percent of all bankruptcy filings in the United States are the direct result of excessive medical expenses.[2]*

- *Health care spending in the United States is more than $1.8 trillion, which is more than four times the amount spent on national defense and almost forty times the amount spent on homeland security.[3]*

- *Although nearly 45 million Americans are uninsured, the United States spends more on health care than other industrialized nations which provide health insurance to all their citizens.[4] In 2003, the United States spent 15.3 percent of its Gross Domestic Product (GDP) on health care. It is projected that the percentage will reach 18.7 percent in 10 years.[5] By contrast, universal health systems in other countries consume much less of their GDP: Canada - 8.4 percent; Sweden - 9.1 percent; Germany - 8.2 percent; Japan - 6.8 percent; United Kingdom - 6.2 percent.[6]*

- *According to the Kaiser Family Foundation and the Health Research and Educational Trust, premiums for employer-sponsored health insurance in the US have risen five times faster than workers' earnings since 2000.[7]*

In fact, most people are shocked to find out that Starbucks Coffee spends more money on health care costs than they do on coffee, and General Motors spends more on health care costs than they do on steel![8]

• *Experts predict retiring elderly couples will need $200,000 in savings just to pay for the most basic medical coverage.[9] Many others believe that this figure is conservative and that $300,000 may be a more realistic number.*

The overall cost of health care—everything from hospital and doctor bills to the cost of pharmaceuticals, medical equipment, insurance, nursing homes, and home health care—doubled from 1993 to 2004, according to a report from the Centers for Medicare and Medicaid Services. In 2004, the nation spent almost $140 billion more for health care than the year before. In fact, more than 15 percent of America's Gross Domestic Product is spent on medical care, or $6,280 per person.[10] That means that $15 of every $100 of our economy goes toward covering the cost of being sick. According to the National Coalition on Health Care, the US health care spending is expected to increase at similar levels for the next decade, reaching $4 trillion in 2015, or 20 percent of the GDP![11]

It's important to remember that the money to cover these costs does not come from thin air. It has to come from all of our pockets. We all pay for these costs in the form of increased taxes and increased cost for all of the stuff that we buy on a daily basis. Consider this. Every time you spend:

- *$1.95 at Starbucks for a cup of coffee, approximately $.30 goes to cover medical costs.*
- *$10 for a movie ticket, approximately $1.50 goes to cover medical costs.*
- *$20 for a pizza, approximately $3 goes to cover medical costs.*
- *$50 for a tank of gas, approximately $7.50 goes to cover medical costs.*
- *$250 for an airline ticket, approximately $37.50 goes to cover medical costs.*
- *$1,000 on auto repairs, approximately $150 goes to cover medical costs.*
- *$2,500 on a plasma television, approximately $375 goes to cover medical costs.*
- *$25,000 on a new car, approximately $1,666 goes to cover medical costs.*

When you consider how many things you buy each month, you can see how quickly the cost of health care adds up!

The incredibly high cost of health care in this country could almost be justified if the enormous expense led to better health among the population, but this hasn't been the case. According to a study by the World Health Organization, the United States ranked a pathetic 15th among 25 industrialized nations based on a wide variety of health measures including infant mortality, the percentage of the population who has access to health care, and the incidence of degenerative disease. The United States ranks behind the entire European Union and countries such as Cuba, South Korea, Singapore, Aruba, Greece, and the Czech Republic.[12]

To make matters worse, the current state of our medicine-based health care system actually contributes to an increase in disease and disability! There is a lot of talk about the devastation of AIDS, which claims the lives of less than 20,000 people per year, according to the Centers for Disease Control (CDC).[99] Yet 199,000 people die unnecessarily from medical care every year, according to a recent article published in the *Journal of the American Medical Association (JAMA)*.[12] In the *JAMA* article, Dr. Barbara Starfield of the Johns Hopkins School of Hygiene and Public Health listed the negative health effects of the US health care system itself, including:

- *$77 billion in unnecessary costs*
- *116 million unnecessary physician visits*
- *77 million unnecessary prescriptions*
- *17 million unnecessary emergency department visits*
- *8 million unnecessary hospitalizations*
- *3 million unnecessary long-term hospital admissions*
- *199,000 unnecessary deaths*
- *20,000 deaths per year from other errors in hospitals*
- *12,000 deaths per year from unnecessary surgery*
- *7,000 deaths per year from medication errors in hospitals*

Many experts, including those from the Food and Drug Administration (FDA), agree that these statistics are a conservative estimate because of the "culture of secrecy" regarding medical error and the enormous malpractice risk that goes along with admitting error. The incredible cost and less than optimal outcome in modern health care occur because we are spending too much money in the wrong place. We have focused far too much attention on exciting new drugs and therapies in the belief that they will lead to better health. But they have not. In fact, they have only served to divert our attention away from the very thing that can help us avoid developing most disease in the first place: living a lifestyle that promotes wellness. That is not to take anything away from the incredible advances that medical research has brought to the treatment of disease. What our country needs, however, is not more medicine, but rather more people who are less sick.

Bankrupting Americans

The high cost of health care and the associated costs of being ill are responsible for half of all personal bankruptcies in this country, according to a study published by the journal *Health Affairs*. This was confirmed by an independent study done by Harvard University. This is true even though most of those filing for bankruptcy had health insurance when they first became sick! But because they either lost their coverage or because they had to pay for expensive treatments not covered by their policy, these people were left financially unprotected.

According to the Harvard study, most people filing for bankruptcy due to medical costs were middle class; 56 percent were homeowners, and 56 percent had attended some college. In some cases, the family's breadwinner was forced to take time off of work, which caused a loss of income and job-based health insurance, compounding the problem.[2]

According to experts in the field, there are several reasons for this trend. Many employers no longer offer a full range of health care benefits, and most now require employees to pay more for coverage out of pocket, or else costs are passed on to employees in the form of policies with higher deductibles.

With co-payments, requirements to pay certain percentages of medical bills, and services that simply aren't covered, even people with insurance have a hard time coming up with the burdensome out-of-pocket health care expenses, and they wind up in debt. A significant percentage of those turn to the bankruptcy courts for relief.

As quoted from a recent article, Jeff Morris, resident scholar at the American Bankruptcy Institute says, "There is a trend toward insurance being viewed as sort of catastrophic protection.... The problem, of course, is it doesn't take a lot of hours at a hospital to generate a bill that is very difficult to pay."

Other health care and social science professionals were interviewed for that same article, and they agree. "I think the message that we take away is, really, nobody is safe in our country. Short of (Microsoft Chairman) Bill Gates, if you're sick enough long enough, you're likely to be financially ruined," cautions Dr. David Himmelstein, an associate professor of medicine at Harvard Medical School, "We're all one serious illness away from bankruptcy." Carol Pryor, a senior policy analyst at The Access Project in Boston, has studied the issue of medical debt and its numerous affects on people's lives, and says that the problem is only likely to escalate due to ever-increasing premiums, deductibles, and co-insurance payments.

The Harvard University study mentioned earlier concluded that financial hardship caused by medical bills affects everyone, not just the uninsured. According to a recent interview with Dr. Steffie Woolhandler, a Harvard associate medical professor and one of the study's authors, "Even the best policies in this country have so many loopholes, it's easy to build up thousands of dollars in expenses."

Even for those in the work force who have insurance, retirement will offer new challenges for maintaining health insurance coverage and for paying for health care. Acting now to promote better health and to prevent disease will pay dividends later in life.

What Is Creating the Health Care Crisis?

According to the Kaiser Family Foundation, the three biggest expenses that we all incur due to America's unhealthy lifestyle are increased costs in hospital care, physician and clinical services, and prescription drugs. It is important to remember that these costs are not the cause of the health care crisis in our country. They are merely a symptom of the problem; a measure of how severe the problem has become.

Hospital Care

Hospital care accounts for the largest percent of health care spending—about one-third of the national health care costs. In recent years, these costs have increased dramatically. "It's not unusual for a hospital's billed charges to increase 25 to 30 percent in one year," says John Bauerlein, senior partner at Milliman USA, a firm that tracks health care spending.

But even more important than the increase in price for services provided is the fact that more people are having to be hospitalized for being sick! According to a report from the American Hospital Association, the most important source of growth was volume—more people using more hospital services. In fact, the total national spending on hospital care rose a whopping $84 billion in just the four years between 1997 and 2001—more than half of that increase was simply from more people being sick.[13]

Physician and Clinical Services

Next on the list of the biggest expenses is physician and clinical services, which makes up about 22 percent of our total health care costs.[14] This includes all the times that we go to see a doctor but we aren't admitted to the hospital. Just like with the increase in utilization of hospital care, the majority of the increase in physician and clinical services is also due to an increase in the demand for services. More people are sick.

Prescription Drugs

Another of the major contributors to rising health care costs is the price of prescription medications and our enormous appetites for these drugs. Americans comprise only five percent of the entire world's population, yet we consume one-half of all the prescription drugs manufactured world-wide—more than three billion prescriptions each year. Five out of six persons 65 and older are taking at least one medication, and almost half the elderly take three or more, according to the US Department of Health and Human Services' annual check-up on Americans' health. Drug expenditures have been the fastest growing segment of health care spending in this country, rising by more than 15 percent every year since 1998.[14]

To put this in perspective, Pulitzer Prize winning journalists Donald Bartlett and James Steele from the *New York Times* write, "In 2002, New York-based Pfizer Inc., the world's largest drug company, reported return on sales of 28.4 percent. That was two and a half times better than the 10.7 percent return of General Electric Company, perennially ranked as America's best-managed business. It was nearly nine times better than the 3.3 percent return of Wal-Mart Stores, the country's largest and best-run retailer. And it was nearly thirty-two times better than the 0.9 percent of General Motors Corporation, America's largest car manufacturer."[15]

The pharmaceutical industry has done a masterful job at convincing people that drugs are intended to cure disease and improve people's lives. But if prescription drugs were the answer to health, then we would have the healthiest nation in the world. However, in spite of our immense drug consumption, the general population is getting heavier, the rates of diabetes, heart disease, and cancer are rising, and we have one of the highest infant mortality rates in the civilized world.

This severe over-reliance on drugs is hastening the death and disability of most of the public. People believe they are "doing something" about their health issues by taking drugs when the underlying challenges—what caused the disease in the first place—are actually being ignored and therefore left to fester. Simultaneously, of course, the revenues of the drug industry continue to increase, meaning ever-fatter checks for all who are directly and indirectly on their payroll and ever-more money spent on marketing and lobbying efforts.

And those marketing and lobbying efforts are worth it. The top selling drugs are consistently manufactured by the drug companies who invest the most on marketing. Lobbying efforts have been so effective that Congress now allows pharmaceutical companies to charge Medicare whatever they want: Congress willingly forfeited its right to negotiate drug prices for Medicare recipients.

The pharmaceutical industry continues to do whatever it can to protect its profits by prohibiting importation of drugs from foreign countries, including Canada, claiming that importation of drugs may be dangerous. When asked why Canada is able to receive such favorable rates compared to America, they explain that Canada has negotiated better rates and that it is America's duty to continue paying such exorbitant fees for supposedly life-saving medications. After all, the pharmaceutical industry argues, they would not be able to afford to continue research and development efforts to search for the next miracle cure. Their emotional appeal to the public has worked and so have their vast lobbying efforts. But if you know better, you can help stop the insanity, help save money, and help save lives.

It is certainly fair to say that there are times when traditional medicine can do amazing things, especially in treating trauma and infectious disease. America has the world's foremost experts at high-tech interventions and there are many well-intentioned, honest medical professionals. But for promoting health, traditional medicine is ineffective and extraordinarily expensive. As wellness expert Dr. Joe Mercola states, "It is indisputable that our current system has enormous benefit and value in the treatment of acute medical emergencies that require the use of trauma centers, skilled surgeons, and intensive care units to help repair us when we are injured. When this system is applied to chronic degenerative health conditions that comprise more than 95 percent of the health problems, it becomes a miserable failure."

Soon, this brewing health care crisis will be worsened by a flood of retiring Baby Boomers whose medical expenses, if current trends continue, will be large enough to bankrupt the country. The conventional medical paradigm has been a destructive influence in our culture, promoting disease by pinning all focus on treatments to combat the symptoms of existing illness while virtually ignoring prevention and wellness.

Current Health Care Solutions Won't Work

There is no longer any disagreement among policy makers, government officials, corporate executives, and business owners that the cost of health care must be brought under control. But there is much disagreement on how to best address the problem. Price controls, strict budgets, and free market competition have been proposed as solutions. But these "solutions" only focus on rationing the availability of health care to the average person and have no effect on improving the health of the population as a whole.

Most public officials agree that the current employer-based health insurance system has major problems, and that something must be done to help the forty-five million uninsured Americans. What to do about the problem is another matter entirely. President George W. Bush has urged the use of health care savings accounts, and is considering whether to force insurance companies to compete for consumers' business by allowing people to buy insurance across state lines. Former House Speaker Newt Gingrich proposed a plan for a nationwide "re-insurance pool" to evenly distribute health care costs. Another popular suggestion is for the federal government to provide health care coverage for all citizens.

Much debate has centered on this problem with no simple solution in sight. It is obvious to everyone that our current system doesn't work.

We Need More People Less Sick

While all of the numbers are big and impressive, it's important to remember that health care costs are not the cause of the health care crisis. They are merely a measure of how severe the health care crisis really is. The reason why the health care crisis exists is simple: there are too many sick people.

As simple a statement as that is, it communicates a real truth about the source of the problem. Any proposed solution to the health care crisis that does not specifically lead to more people being less sick is doomed to failure. Just like changing seats on the Titanic, it can only, at best, delay the inevitable.

There is an old saying that nothing good in life comes free. This is true when it comes to your body as well. Living a wellness lifestyle requires you to be a proactive agent for your body. You need to treat it well and not wait until you hurt before you decide to take care of it. Health is not merely the absence of disease any more than wealth is an absence of poverty. Health is not simply "feeling fine," for we know that problems may progress for years without causing any symptoms whatsoever. For example, heart disease often progresses unnoticed for many years before it rears its ugly head. In fact, the first symptom that many people experience with heart disease is a heart attack or death.

I work hard to get people to understand that it is much better to prevent disease from happening in the first place than try to treat it once it occurs. By creating a state of optimal health within your body, you will feel better, have more energy, and increase your quality of life. You will also reduce your risk of the expense and pain associated with getting hooked into the downward spiral of disease and dependence on more and more prescription medications.

The main ideas that I really want to drive home in this book are: 1) illness causes bankruptcy in every way, 2) most of our health care dollars are spent on expensive treatments for lifestyle-related chronic conditions, 3) each of us has the opportunity to enrich our lives by adopting a wellness lifestyle, and 4) each of us has the responsibility to ourselves and to our country to do our part in solving America's health care crisis by promoting our own well-being.

Each of the book's sixteen chapters covers important topics that are relevant to your health. You will learn how the major diseases—heart disease, cancer, diabetes, and obesity— are largely the consequence of poor lifestyle choices, and you will learn the components of health that will lead to a lifetime of wellness: alignment, nutrition, exercise, healthy thinking and healthy lifestyle habits. Finally, you will learn about the importance of having your own hand-picked wellness team to help you build up a rich reserve of health to carry into your future.

In this book, I want to share with you the best and latest information on wellness so that you can look and feel your very best. It has been my experience that people who are free from chronic pain, who are active, and who feel their best are the people who are also the happiest with themselves, nicest to others, and best able to contribute to their employers, families, and communities. They have the most rewarding relationships and spend the least on medical expenses. It is this combination of factors that makes people RICH.

1

Cardiovascular Disease

L et's begin by learning about cardiovascular disease, by far the most expensive and most common lifestyle-related disease. According to the US Centers for Disease Control (CDC), about 71 million Americans (almost one-fourth of the population) have some form of cardiovascular disease, and about 950,000 Americans die of cardiovascular disease each year: that amounts to one death every 35 seconds. Coronary artery disease, which is a condition where the arteries that feed the heart become clogged, is a leading cause of premature, permanent disability among working adults, costs the US more than $400 billion per year in medical expenses and lost productivity, and is responsible for almost six million hospitalizations each year.[2]

Cardiovascular disease, sometimes called "heart disease," is a blanket term that describes a family of conditions that affect the heart and circulatory system,[1] including hypertension (high blood pressure), atherosclerosis, heart attack, abnormal heart rhythm (arrhythmia), and congestive heart failure. Essentially, any condition that interferes with the normal pumping of the heart or the normal flow of blood falls under the umbrella of cardiovascular disease.

Cardiovascular diseases are often called "silent killers," as they typically progress unnoticed in the body for years before they are discovered. Too often the first sign of cardiovascular disease is sudden death from a heart attack. In fact, the majority of the most serious, life-threatening conditions—cardiovascular disease, cancer, diabetes—have few, if any, recognizable symptoms. It is impossible to gauge how healthy you are simply by how you feel. You can be 24 hours away from death and still feel fine. For this reason, it is very important to have regular checkups with your wellness doctor and not rely merely on how you feel day to day.

The cardiovascular system is also known as the circulatory system. It consists of the heart, which is a muscular pumping device, and a closed system of vessels called arteries, veins, and capillaries. The role of the cardiovascular system in maintaining homeostasis is the transportation of nutrients and oxygen from the digestive system to all of the cells in the body, as well as the transportation of waste and carbon dioxide to be eliminated.

The normal human heart is a strong, muscular pump a little larger than a fist. Each day an average heart beats 100,000 times and pumps about 2,000 gallons of blood. In an average lifetime, the human heart will beat more than 2.5 billion times. The heart pumps blood continuously through the circulatory system. The circulatory system is a network of vessels that carries blood throughout the body. These blood vessels carry oxygen-rich blood from the lungs to all parts of the body.

The network of vessels is so vast that if you were to lay all these vessels end to end, they'd encircle the earth more than twice. The circulating blood brings oxygen and nutrients to all the body's organs and tissues, including the heart itself. It also picks up waste products from the body's cells. These waste products are removed as they're filtered through the kidneys, liver, and lungs.

As long as your cardiovascular system works correctly, your body has an enormous capacity to adapt to just about any external demand. For example, when you begin to exercise, your heart pumps faster and your blood pressure increases in order to supply more oxygen and nutrients to your tissues. When you are cold, your blood vessels constrict in certain areas of the body in an effort to conserve heat. When your body is injured, the blood vessels open up to allow white blood cells to enter the area to fight infection and to speed healing.

The Economic Costs of Cardiovascular Disease

The economic impact of cardiovascular disease on the US health care system grows larger as the population ages. In 2003, the cost of heart disease and stroke was approximately $209 billion for health care expenditures and $142 billion for lost productivity from death and disability. Today, the estimated direct and indirect cost of cardiovascular disease tops $403 billion![3]

Personal Impact

It is tempting when looking at large economic numbers to see them as somehow separate from ourselves, as though the billions of dollars spent on cardiovascular disease will not affect our personal pocketbooks. But the more than $400 billion

Did You Know?

- *An estimated 71 million Americans have one or more forms of cardiovascular disease (CVD).*
- *Cardiovascular disease is responsible for one of every 2.7 deaths.*
- *Since 1900, CVD has been the number one killer in the United States every year except 1918.*
- *Nearly 2,500 Americans die of CVD each day, an average of one death every 35 seconds. CVD claims more lives each year than the next four leading causes of death combined, which are cancer, chronic lower respiratory diseases, accidents, and diabetes mellitus.*

(Source: The American Heart Association Statistics Committee.[3])

annual cost has to be paid by each individual in this country: this translates to $5,520 per year for a family of four! The costs are even higher among those in treatment for cardiovascular disease, who have to pay for prescription drugs and additional doctor visits. Would it be worth changing a few lifestyle habits if it meant that you could have an extra $5,520 per year?[4]

As dramatic as the economic costs of cardiovascular disease are, there are also the quality-of-life costs. Not only does cardiovascular disease shorten your lifespan by almost a decade, but it can also lead to chronic pain and a severe limitation of your daily activities.

Our Personal Health Care Bill
(based on a family of four)

Heart Disease   *$5,520 / year*   *$460 / month*

(Calculated by taking the total health care cost of the disease and dividing it by the total population.)

Current Treatments

Current medical treatments for cardiovascular disease fall into two general categories: drugs and surgery. The drugs include a class of compounds called "statins" that are used for decreasing cholesterol levels, antihypertensives that help reduce blood pressure, and anticoagulants (blood thinners) that are designed to keep the blood from clotting.

Surgical interventions include the coronary bypass, where blood vessels are stripped from the leg and used to help reroute blood flow in the heart; angioplasty, which uses a balloon or laser to force open the arteries around the heart; or open-heart surgery to repair or replace heart valves.

Unfortunately, these treatments are not the answer to the problem of rampant cardiovascular disease. They only help to ameliorate the physical symptoms once heart disease has occurred—often at a considerable cost. The long-term solution to the economic and human hardship resulting from cardiovascular disease is to have more people who are less sick. This is not achieved through more drugs or better surgery, but through a healthier lifestyle.

Lifestyle Solutions

The cardiovascular system is the one that fails most often due to an unhealthy lifestyle. The vast majority of heart disease is completely avoidable by making some simple lifestyle changes—exercise being the most important. The key phrase for your cardiovascular health is "use it or lose it." If you don't exercise and work out your cardiovascular system, you will lose it. Like virtually all forms of physical bankruptcy, heart disease is most often the result of simply not paying attention to managing your health.

According to Alice Lichtenstein, D.Sc., Chair of the American Heart Association's Nutrition Committee and Gershoff Professor at the Friedman School of Nutrition Science and Policy at Tufts University in Boston, "The key message is to focus on long-term, permanent changes in how we eat and live. The best way to lower cardiovascular risk is to combine physical activity with heart-healthy eating habits, coupled with weight control and avoiding tobacco products." In other words, by living a lifestyle of wellness, you can dramatically decrease your risk of developing heart disease.

It may be tempting to believe that doing just one healthy thing will be enough to avoid heart disease. For example, you may hope that if you walk or swim regularly, you can still eat a lot of fatty foods and be safe. Not so. To reduce your risk of a heart attack and other complications, it is vital to make changes that address each area of your lifestyle. You can make the changes gradually, one at a time, but making them is very important.

There are several lifestyle changes that will help you achieve better health. You can implement these changes today to decrease your risk of cardiovascular disease and improve your overall quality of life.

Lifestyle Habits

Quit smoking. Tobacco use increases the risk of heart disease and heart attack. Cigarette smoking promotes atherosclerosis and increases the levels of blood clotting factors, such as fibrinogen. Also, nicotine raises blood pressure, and carbon monoxide reduces the amount of oxygen that blood can carry. Exposure to other people's smoke can increase the risk of heart disease even for nonsmokers.

Limit alcohol consumption. Excessive alcohol use leads to an increase in blood pressure and increases the risk for heart disease. It also increases blood levels of triglycerides which contribute to atherosclerosis.

Maintain a healthy body weight. Being overweight dramatically increases your risk of developing cardiovascular disease. Obesity as a major risk factor for heart disease is even more alarming when you consider that one out of every three Americans is obese. Recent studies have shown that obesity is linked to 280,000 deaths in the United States each year. If you are overweight, reducing your weight by only ten percent can cut your risk of developing heart disease by 50 percent![5]

Spinal Alignment

At first it may seem strange to include a section on spinal alignment in a chapter on heart disease. But, just like every other organ in the body, the heart is controlled by the nervous system—in particular, the nerves that exit the spine in the upper thoracic area.

Whenever there is a misalignment of the bones in the spine—the vertebrae—the nerves that have to wind their way between those vertebrae on the path between the spinal cord and the rest of the body become irritated. This irritation then leads to a disruption in the nerve's ability to communicate correctly with its target. Sometimes the nerve becomes inflamed and fires too much; sometimes it fires too little. In either case, whenever a nerve becomes irritated, the body cannot function correctly.

When it comes to the function of the heart, if any of the nerves exiting the spine in the upper part of the thorax become inflamed, the proper function of the heart and circulatory system can be affected. This is one of the reasons why poor posture of the upper back and neck can have such a destructive effect on your health, and why people who sit at desks all day have an increased risk of indigestion and heart disease. Misaligned vertebrae in the upper back may not be the primary cause of heart disease, but they certainly can contribute to a loss of normal heart function.

Exercise

According to the *US Surgeon General's Report on Physical Activity and Health*, inactive people are nearly twice as likely to develop heart disease as those who are more active. This is true even if they have no other conditions or habits that increase the risk of heart disease. Lack of physical activity contributes to a variety of illnesses, leading to more visits to the doctor, more hospitalizations, and more use of medicines.

The good news is that physical activity can protect your heart in a number of important ways. Moreover, to get the benefits of exercise, you don't need to be able to run a marathon. Regular activity—something as simple as a brisk 30-minute walk each day—can help you reduce your risk of heart disease.

Nutrition

Poor nutrition is one of the major contributors to the development of heart disease. The average American consumes too many calories, far too much fat, way too much sugar, and not nearly enough fresh fruits and vegetables. Poor nutrition, especially when combined with stress, leads to a condition of chronic inflammation in the body. It is this chronic inflammation that causes cardiovascular disease to emerge.

A healthy diet is among the best weapons you have to fight cardiovascular disease. It's not as hard as you may think! Remember, it is the overall pattern of your eating choices that counts. Good nutrition means eating a variety of foods, moderating your intake of certain foods and drinks, and controlling the amount of food and calories you eat. It also means making sure that you get enough of the right kind of foods, such as antioxidant-rich fruits and vegetables.

Healthy Thinking

Stress is linked to heart disease in a number of ways. Research shows that the most commonly reported "trigger" for a heart attack is an emotionally upsetting event, particularly one involving anger. Some common ways of coping with stress, such as overeating, heavy drinking, and smoking, are clearly bad for your heart. In order to reduce your risk of cardiovascular disease, it is important to learn how to positively reduce stress in your life. You will learn some simple techniques for reducing stress later on in this book.

2

Cancer

C ancer is currently the second leading cause of death in the United States. According to the American Cancer Society (ACS), more than half a million Americans died of cancer in 2004: that is more than 1,500 people a day. One of every four deaths in America is from cancer, and over two million new cases of cancer will be diagnosed this year. According to the World Health Organization, the number of new cancer cases worldwide is expected to increase by fifty percent over the next twenty years, partly because more nations are adopting unhealthy Western habits.

So why does cancer develop? Much like a pack of wolves pursuing a herd of elk, or a lion stalking a group of gazelles, cancer looks for the weakest cells in the body to attack. Wherever the body is weakened by stress, toxins, poor nutrition, or lack of exercise, cancer has a better chance of getting a foothold. It is true that some people have a genetic predisposition to certain types of cancer, particularly breast cancer, but the single most important factor that determines whether someone will develop cancer is lifestyle.

The body is made up of many types of cells. Normally, cells grow and divide to produce more cells as they are needed to keep the body healthy. Sometimes, this orderly process goes wrong. New cells form where the body does not need them, and old cells do not die when they should. Cancer is a disease where cells in the body reproduce abnormally, creating an excessive growth of mutated cells that, over time, interfere with normal body function.

As doctors, scientists, and researchers know, people experience abnormal cell growth every day; but the innate intelligence of the body is able to correct that abnormal growth and stabilize the negative effects through the healthy function of the immune system.

Tobacco use, physical inactivity, obesity, and poor nutrition are among the major causes of cancer and other diseases in the United States. The American Cancer Society estimates that in 2006, more than 170,000 cancer deaths will be caused by tobacco use alone. In addition, scientists estimate that approximately one-third of the 564,830 cancer deaths expected to occur in 2006 will be related to poor nutrition, physical inactivity, and excessive weight.[1-3]

Another leading cause of cancer is exposure to industrial toxins. According to the Environmental Protection Agency's (EPA) *Toxic Release Inventory*, every year a combined two million tons of more than 10,000 industrial chemicals are released into the environment. Out of these, less than two percent have been thoroughly studied for their potential toxic effects on humans. These chemicals make their way into your body through the water you drink, the food you eat, and the air you breathe; if they accumulate in your body, they will dramatically increase your risk of cancer. This is a primary reason why many people spend extra money to buy "organic" foods which are grown without the use of industrial chemicals.

To a large extent, these causes of cancer are preventable. Although we cannot control our genes and we cannot always control the chemicals to which we get exposed in the environment, we always have a choice in the care we take of our bodies: what foods we eat, whether we exercise, whether we receive routine health care, and how much clean water we drink.

Did You Know?

- *More than 1.3 million people in the United States were diagnosed with cancer in 2003.[4]*
- *Approximately one-third of cancer deaths are related to poor nutrition, physical inactivity, and excessive weight.[1-3]*
- *According to the American Cancer Society (ACS), more than half a million Americans died of cancer in 2004: that is more than 1,500 people a day.[4]*

The Economic Costs of Cancer

More than 1.3 million people in the United States were diagnosed with cancer in 2003, and the incidence of cancer continues to increase: that ranks cancer among the most significant contributors of health care spending in the United States. In 2002, the National Institutes of Health estimated that cancer cost this country $60.9 billion in direct medical costs and $110.7 billion in indirect and mortality costs.[4] By 2004, these costs had jumped to $74 billion in direct medical costs and $135 billion in indirect costs due to illness: a total of $210 billion![5]

Personal Impact

Just as with all other health care expenses in this country, the money to pay for these cancer costs has to come from somewhere. A portion of it comes right out of your pocket in the form of taxes, insurance premiums, co-payments, and higher prices on items we buy every day. How much does our cancer crisis cost you? Every man, woman, and child in this country has to contribute $719 each year—a cost of almost $3,000 for a family of four. That's a lot of money.

As dramatic as the economic costs of cancer are, there are also the quality-of-life costs. Many of the therapies for cancer are themselves so physically debilitating that patients often cannot function; they are unable to work for extended periods of time and remain very sick. Plus, some treatments in use are so invasive and toxic they carry their own long-term negative effects for the patient's health.

Our Personal Health Care Bill
(based on a family of four)

Heart Disease	*$5,520 / year*	*$460 / month*
Cancer	*$2,876 / year*	*$240 / month*

*(Calculated by taking the total health care cost of these diseases
and dividing it by the total population.)*

Current Treatments

Traditional medical therapy for cancer may include surgery, radiation therapy, chemotherapy, and hormone therapy. Many doctors use a combination of methods, depending on the type and location of the cancer.

While all of these therapies have been used with varying degrees of success, none of them really addresses the central problem associated with cancer—the fact that too many people get it in the first place. The ultimate solution to the health care crisis in this country is to have more people less sick. I have said it before because it is the central concept of this book. Too often we become so enamored with our ability to treat disease with very creative treatments and expensive high-tech equipment that we lose sight of the fact that no treatment can ever be as effective as prevention. We cannot "treat" our way out of our personal and national health care crisis. We must find solutions aimed at the source of the problem.

Lifestyle Solutions

Just as with cardiovascular disease, there are lifestyle changes you can implement today to decrease your risk of developing cancer and to improve your overall quality of life.

Lifestyle Habits

Don't use tobacco. All types of tobacco put you on a collision course with cancer. Rejecting tobacco is one of the most important health decisions you can make. Avoiding tobacco in any form significantly reduces your risk of several cancers, including cancer of the lung, esophagus, mouth, bladder, kidneys, pancreas, and stomach.

In the United States, smoking is responsible for about 90 percent of all cases of lung cancer—the leading cause of cancer death in both men and women. Every time you smoke a cigarette, you inhale more than 60 substances that can cause your cells to become cancerous. Even if you don't smoke, secondhand smoke is also very dangerous. In fact, about 3,000 nonsmokers die of lung cancer every year because of secondhand smoke.[1]

Protect yourself from the sun. Skin cancer is one of the most common forms of cancer and is also one of the most preventable. The most common cause of skin cancer is over-exposure to ultraviolet (UV) radiation from the sun or from tanning beds. Although skin cancer is one of the easier forms of cancer to treat as long as it is discovered early, it is much better to reduce your risk of developing it in the first place. Here are a few things that you can do to reduce your risk of skin cancer:

- *Avoid overexposing your skin to direct sunlight during the peak UV radiation hours, usually between 10:00 a.m. and 4:00 p.m.*
- *If you are going to be outside, wear sunscreen and cover exposed areas with light-colored, loose-fitting clothing.*
- *Avoid using indoor tanning beds or sunlamps, as these can damage your skin as much as the sun can.*

Maintain a Healthy Weight

The American Cancer Society was one of the first national organizations to call attention to the relationship between obesity and cancer. In 2003, they released the most comprehensive study to date on the relationship between excess body weight and cancer mortality.[6] They found that the more overweight an individual is, the greater that person's risk of dying from many different types of cancer—esophageal, stomach, breast, colorectal, liver, gallbladder, pancreatic, prostate, kidney, lymphoma, multiple myeloma, and leukemia.[7]

Spinal Alignment

Cancer has sometimes been described as a disease of a confused immune system. You see, cancerous cells develop in everyone's body just about every day. But our immune system knows how to recognize a cell that is unhealthy and eliminate it. If the immune system becomes compromised in some way, due to a major long-term illness or chronic stress, it loses some of its ability to find cancer cells. Believe it or not, our central nervous system plays a major role in the function of our immune system. This is why people are more likely to get sick or develop cancer when they experience severe or long-term stress.

As discussed in the last chapter on heart disease, whenever a misaligned spine compromises the nervous system, one of the first measurable changes that occurs in the body is a suppression of immune function. In fact, studies have shown that there are measurable improvements in immune function within minutes after a spinal adjustment, as measured by antibodies in the saliva.

In order to minimize your risk of developing cancer, it is necessary to do whatever you can to keep your immune system working properly. One way to do this is to remove any source of irritation by keeping your spine healthy and aligned.

Exercise

Exercising regularly also plays an important role in preventing cancer. Obesity may be a risk factor for cancer of the prostate, colon, rectum, uterus, ovaries, and breast. Physical activity can help you avoid obesity by controlling your weight.

Try to be physically active for 30 minutes or more on most days of the week. These periods of exercise can include such low-key activities as brisk walking, raking the yard, or even ballroom dancing.

Nutrition

Large portion sizes and calorie-dense foods are used extensively to market foods in restaurants and supermarkets. Changes in urban design and land use have reduced opportunities for physical activity. Scientific evidence suggests that about one-third of the cancer deaths that occur in the US each year are due to nutrition and physical activity factors, including obesity.[2,4]

To dramatically reduce your chances of developing cancer, be sure to eat five or more servings of fruits and vegetables each day. Also eat other foods from plant sources, such as whole grains and beans, several times a day. Green and dark yellow vegetables, legumes, soybean products, and cruciferous vegetables—such as broccoli, Brussels sprouts, and cabbage— are excellent choices. Diets high in fruits and vegetables are associated with a lower risk of cancers of the mouth and pharynx, esophagus, lung, stomach, colon, and rectum.[7]

Whenever possible, eat lighter and leaner by choosing fewer high-fat foods. High-fat diets may increase your risk of cancer of the prostate, colon, rectum, and uterus.

Healthy Thinking

It has been long known that stress contributes to the development of heart disease. Recent research has shown that heightened stress can also increase a person's susceptibility to cancer or worsen the prognosis of an existing cancer. Studies have shown that chronic and acute stressors, including surgery and social disruptions, appear to promote tumor growth. This makes sense when you think about it. Since cancer cells tend to attack the weak cells in the body, and we know that stress can weaken these cells, then it should follow that stress makes the body more susceptible to developing cancer.

So just as in the case of heart disease, it is critical to learn to minimize the negative effects of stress and develop healthy thinking habits.

3

Diabetes

Almost everyone knows someone who has diabetes. In fact, from 1980 through 2004, the total number of Americans with diabetes more than doubled.[1] An estimated 18.2 million people in the United States—about six percent of the entire population—have diabetes, a serious, lifelong condition. Of those, about six million people have not yet been diagnosed.

Diabetes is a condition that occurs when the body has lost its ability to regulate the levels of glucose (sugar) in the bloodstream. This is usually due to some interruption in the production of insulin, the hormone that lowers blood sugar levels. The ability to regulate glucose is vital to the functioning of your entire system. Since all of the organs of the body rely on a steady supply of glucose in order to function correctly, any disruption in blood sugar levels can have dire consequences.

There are two major types of diabetes: Type 1 (also called "juvenile diabetes") and Type 2 (also called "adult-onset diabetes"). Type 1 diabetes usually strikes children and young adults, although the disease can occur at any age. In Type 1 diabetes, beta cells in the pancreas, the cells in the body that make insulin, simply do not function. So, in order to manage their blood sugar levels, people with Type 1 diabetes must inject insulin directly into their body or have it delivered by a small pump. Type 1 diabetes accounts for five to ten percent of all diagnosed cases of diabetes.[1]

By far, the more common type of diabetes is Type 2: it accounts for about 90 to 95 percent of all diagnosed cases of diabetes. Type 2 diabetes usually begins as "insulin resistance," a disorder in which the cells of the body lose their ability to use insulin properly. This, in turn, places extra demands upon the pancreas, which must release more insulin to make up for the loss of normal insulin action. Over time, the pancreas becomes exhausted and gradually loses its ability to produce insulin at all. But why would the body's cells develop insulin resistance in the first place? Aging and family history are factors, but Type 2 diabetes is also widely associated with lifestyle habits such as lack of exercise, obesity, poor diet, and stress.[1]

In 2000, diabetes ranked as the sixth leading cause of death in the United States, but this figure may actually underestimate the disease's impact. Diabetes is not always noted as the underlying cause of death on a death certificate: about 65 percent of the deaths among those with diabetes are attributed to heart disease and stroke. Moreover, incidence of the disease is expected to spread as our population ages and grows increasingly overweight and sedentary.

Diabetes is also one of the leading causes of disability in America. The long-term complications of diabetes can affect almost every part of the body, often leading to blindness, heart and blood vessel disease, stroke, kidney failure, amputations, and nerve damage. Uncontrolled diabetes can complicate

---

Did You Know?

- *Approximately 798,000 new cases of diabetes are diagnosed annually in the United States.*
- *12,000 new cases of blindness annually in the United States are due to diabetes.*
- *Diabetes can be a deadly disease: over 200,000 people die each year of diabetes-related complications.*
- *Cardiovascular disease is the most costly complication of diabetes, accounting for more than $17.6 billion of the $91.8 billion annual direct medical costs for diabetes in 2002.*
- *In 2002, diabetes accounted for a loss of nearly 88 million disability days and resulted in 176,000 cases of permanent disability, at a cost of $7.5 billion.*

(Source: Centers for Disease Control (CDC), American Diabetes Association.[2])

pregnancy, and birth defects are more common in babies born to women with diabetes.

In addition, the American Diabetes Association estimates that nearly six million Americans are currently living with undiagnosed diabetes. "It is often not until their eyes, nerves, and kidneys fail, or they have a heart attack or a stroke, that they discover that they have been living with this chronic disease," says Robert Sherwin, the President of the American Diabetes Association. Unfortunately, many people have diabetes for years before symptoms show or before it is diagnosed, and during that time the disease is taking its toll, unchecked, upon the body.

The Economic Costs of Diabetes

Diabetes alone represents 11 percent of the United States health care expenditure. People with diabetes have medical expenditures 2.4 times higher than they would if they did not have diabetes. One out of every ten health care dollars spent in the United States is spent on diabetes and its complications.[2]

According to the CDC, diabetes cost the United States $132 billion in 2002. This includes the direct medical costs of diabetes care, including hospitalizations, medical care, and treatment supplies, and also the indirect costs, such as disability payments, time lost from work, and premature death. Over the next ten years, with incidence of diabetes continually on the rise, our diabetes bill will continue to increase.[3]

Personal Impact

As with all other health care expenses in this country, the money to pay for the costs associated with diabetes has to come from somewhere. You guessed it. It comes right out of your pocket, not only in insurance premiums and co-payments, but also in taxes and in higher prices on consumer items. How much does the nation's diabetes epidemic cost you? Every man, woman, and child in this country has to contribute $452 each year—a cost of $1,808 for a family of four. And for those afflicted with diabetes, annual personal expenses to pay for medications, doctor visits, and lost wages are increased by several thousand dollars per year. That's a lot of money.

We can see our family's health care bill increasing, but how do we measure the quality-of-life costs to those affected by diabetes? These uncountable costs can be staggering. Diabetes leads to blindness, kidney failure, neuropathies, amputated limbs,

---

Our Personal Health Care Bill
(based on a family of four)

Heart Disease	*$5,520 / year*	*$460 / month*
Cancer	*$2,876 / year*	*$240 / month*
Diabetes	*$1,808 / year*	*$151 / month*

(Calculated by taking the total health care cost of these diseases and dividing it by the total population.)

and a shortened life span. Even the day-to-day maintenance of the disease can be stressful: diabetes sufferers must constantly monitor their blood sugar and ensure they receive their daily medications.

Current Treatments

The most common forms of medical treatment for diabetes include the use of insulin injections and oral medications to lower blood sugar. While these treatment methods can be very useful in managing diabetes once it occurs, they do little to avert the development of the disease. It is impossible to medicate our way out of the epidemic of diabetes in this country. The true solution lies in our ability to prevent disease, rather than our ability to "fix" or manage it. In other words, the answer is to have more people who are less sick!

Lifestyle Solutions

Many, if not most, cases of diabetes are the result of an unhealthy lifestyle. Habits such as consuming too much sugar, living with too much stress, getting only poor nutrition, being overweight, and not getting enough exercise can lead directly to the development of Type 2 diabetes. This is actually good news: it means we have the power to influence our health by our own lifestyle choices. A recently completed Diabetes Prevention Program study by the American Diabetes

Association conclusively showed that by making changes in diet and increasing physical activity, people with "pre-diabetes" (when blood sugar levels are higher than normal but not yet in the diabetic range) can prevent the development of Type 2 diabetes—they may even be able to return their blood glucose levels to the normal range. Just 30 minutes a day of moderate physical activity, coupled with a five to ten percent reduction in body weight, produced a 58 percent reduction in diabetes![4]

Maintain a Healthy Weight

Obesity is one of the major contributors to the development of diabetes. In fact, according to the American Diabetes Association, 90 percent of all people who are diagnosed with diabetes are overweight. With 61 percent of the US adult population considered to be overweight or obese, it is easy to see how diabetes has become such a problem. According to a study of the American Diabetes Association, even a five to ten percent reduction in body weight can result in a tremendous reduction in the risk or severity of diabetes. For most people, that is only a loss of 10-20 pounds.

Exercise

Physical activity can lower your blood sugar (glucose) and help insulin work better for your body. Your body is then less susceptible to the development of diabetes. Regular exercise also helps lower blood pressure and cholesterol levels, thereby reducing your risk of heart disease and stroke. Exercise relieves stress and strengthens your heart, muscles, and bones; it improves your blood circulation, and keeps your joints flexible. If you're trying to lose weight, a combination of physical activity and wise food choices can help you reach your target weight and maintain it. All of these benefits can be yours even if you haven't been very active before.

Nutrition

Eating habits contribute significantly to the current epidemic of diabetes. If you go back in history, people never before had access to the endless stream of soft drinks, candy bars, cookies, muffins, and other starchy foods, as we do today. In fact, our ancestors ate very little grain. Only very recently did people begin to eat so many carbohydrates and sugars.

Eating a lot of carbohydrates every day puts stress on the pancreas, which must work harder to maintain a stable blood sugar level. Over time, the pancreas becomes worn out and can no longer keep up with all the carbohydrates that are coming into your system. When this happens, diabetes results.

4

Chronic Pain

The word "pain" comes from the Latin *poena* meaning a fine, a penalty. You can think about pain as the primary way that the body lets you know that something is wrong and needs your attention. In this way, you can think about the word "pain" as an acronym for Pay Attention Inside Now. Doctors make a distinction between "acute pain" and "chronic pain." Acute pain is a normal short-term sensation that is experienced when a part of the body is injured. With acute pain, once the pain subsides, there is no recurrence, unless there is a re-injury to the area. But chronic pain is different.

Chronic pain is not a single entity but varies in origin and characteristics. It may have been caused by an initial injury—a sprained back, whiplash, or sports injury—or some organic disorder—arthritis, cancer, or ear infection—but these are not always necessary for a chronic pain syndrome to appear. Chronic pain, by definition, persists for a long period of time (more than three to six months) and may recur without any identifiable reason. Many older adults suffer from chronic pain, but it should not be classified as merely a result of aging. In fact, the majority of chronic pain conditions occur in people between the ages of 24 and 64.[1]

The common manifestations of acute or chronic pain include head pain, joint pain, back pain, neck pain, burning arm or leg pain, nerve pain, chest pain, abdominal pain, and pain associated with cancer.[2] In this chapter, we will focus on the three most common types of chronic pain: arthritis, neck and back pain, and headaches.

Arthritis

The term "arthritis" literally means "joint inflammation." An estimated 43 million people in the United States suffer from arthritis, or other rheumatic conditions, and this number is expected to reach 60 million by the year 2020.[3] Arthritic disorders are characterized by joint pain in the spine and extremities; other inflammatory diseases which affect the body's soft tissues include tendonitis and bursitis.

Of the many different types of arthritis, only a small percentage tends to cause chronic pain. When these do strike, however, the results can be disabling. Let's examine the three most common forms of arthritis that can lead to chronic pain: osteoarthritis, ankylosing spondylitis, and rheumatoid arthritis.

Osteoarthritis

Osteoarthritis is the most common type of arthritis, affecting an estimated 21 million adults in the United States.[4] It is a chronic disease that leads to the deterioration of your joint cartilage (the soft pads of cushioning between the bones in each of your joints), as well as the formation of abnormal bone spurs. Osteoarthritis primarily affects the weight-bearing joints, such as the knees, hips, and spine. When osteoarthritis affects the lower back, disc degeneration is often the result.

Ankylosing Spondylitis

Ankylosing spondylitis tends to affect people—primarily men—in late adolescence or early adulthood. Ankylosing spondylitis (AS) leads to the inflammation and calcification (hardening) of the long, tough ligament that helps to stabilize the spine, called the "anterior longitudinal ligament." AS causes a gradual, progressive loss of mobility in the spine and episodes of considerable back pain. AS may also affect the hips, shoulders, and knees as the tendons and ligaments around the bones and joints become inflamed.[5]

Rheumatoid Arthritis

Rheumatoid arthritis (RA) is an inflammatory disease of the synovium, or the tissue that encapsulates each of your joints. Inflammation of the synovium with RA results in pain, stiffness, swelling, and loss of function of the joints. In later stages of the disease, the spine may also be affected, though symptoms most commonly manifest in the neck. Rheumatoid arthritis generally occurs in a symmetrical pattern. This means that if one knee or hand is involved, the other one is also. Those who suffer from RA often experience fatigue, occasional fever, and a general sense of not feeling well.

Neck and Back Pain

Back pain is one of the most significant health problems facing Americans: 85 percent of all people will experience back pain at some time in their lives. Disability due to chronic low back pain is the most expensive benign condition that is medically treated in industrialized countries. Back pain is the second most common reason for visits to the doctor's office, outnumbered only by upper-respiratory infections. In fact, the National Institutes of Health reports that back pain is the most frequent cause of activity limitation in people less than 45 years of age; after 45, it is still the third leading cause of disability. The pain and disability associated with low back disc herniations alone costs the health care system more than $50 billion a year.[6]

Here we will discuss several of the major conditions that can lead to chronic neck and back pain: misalignments in the spine, disc herniations, and stress.

Misalignments in the Spine

Whenever there is a disruption in the normal movement or position of the vertebrae in your spine, with time it will result in inflammation and pain. These disruptions often occur at the transitional areas between the head and neck, neck and upper back, and lower spine and sacrum, or tailbone. Subtle dislocations of the vertebrae, called subluxations, can lead to spinal degeneration and debilitating pain. Fortunately, subluxations are easily managed by spinal adjustments, and often a significant reduction in pain is experienced almost immediately after care.

Disc Herniations

A disc herniation occurs when there is a protruding bulge on the exposed surface of a disc. Contrary to popular belief, a herniated disc does not automatically mean that you are going to suffer from low back pain. In fact, one study found that almost half of all adults have at least one bulging or herniated disc, many without experiencing any discomfort. However, if the herniation is significant enough to compress tissues surrounding the spine, it can be a source of intense and debilitating pain that frequently radiates to other areas of the body. Unfortunately, once a disc herniates, it rarely, if ever, completely heals. Further deterioration can often be avoided through regular spinal care, but a complete recovery is much less common.

Stress

Whenever you become stressed, your body responds by increasing your blood pressure and heart rate, flooding your body with stress hormones, and tightening up your muscles. When you are stressed much of the time, chronic tension causes your muscles to become sore, weak, and loaded with trigger points. If you experience a great deal of pain associated with stress, it is important to practice some form of relaxation, such as deep breathing, or even exercise. This will help to reduce tension in your muscles and decrease pain.

Headaches

Headaches affect just about everyone at some point and can present themselves in many different ways. Headache pain may concentrate in one part of the head or behind the eyes, or it may become a pounding sensation inside the whole head; it may be accompanied by nausea, or it may not. The pain itself may be dull or sharp, and it may last anywhere from a few minutes to a few days. Fortunately, very few headaches have serious underlying causes, but those that do require urgent medical attention.

Although headaches can be due to a wide variety of causes, such as drug reactions, temporomandibular joint dysfunction (TMJ), tightness in the neck muscles, low blood sugar, high blood pressure, spinal misalignments, stress, and fatigue, the majority of recurrent headaches are of two types: tension headaches (also called cervicogenic headaches) and migraine headaches. There is a third, less common, type of headache called a cluster headache that is a cousin to the migraine. Here we take a closer look at each of these three types of headaches.

Tension Headaches

Tension headaches are the most common, accounting for more than 75 percent of all headaches. Most people describe a tension headache as a constant, dull, achy feeling on one or both sides of the head, or as a tight band or dull ache around the head or behind the eyes. This may last from 30 minutes to several days. These headaches usually begin gradually, and tend to emerge in the middle or toward the end of the day. Tension headaches are often the result of stress or bad posture, which aggravates the spine and muscles in the upper back and neck.[7]

Migraine Headaches

Each year, about 25 million people in the US experience migraine headaches; about 75 percent are women. Migraines are intense, pounding headaches caused by the constriction and then over-dilation of blood vessels in the brain. They can last from as little as a few hours to as long as a few days. Many of those who suffer from migraines experience a visual symptom called an "aura" just prior to an attack: they may see flashing lights or notice their surroundings take on a dream-like appearance.

For those who are predisposed to them, a number of things can trigger a migraine: lack of sleep, stress, flickering lights, even strong odors. Migraines are often associated with nausea and sensitivity to light or noise.[7]

Cluster Headaches

Cluster headaches are typically excruciating headaches of very short duration, usually felt on one side of the head behind the eyes. Cluster headaches affect about one million people in the United States and, unlike migraines, are much more common in men. This is the only type of headache that tends to occur at night. The reason they are called 'cluster' headaches is that they tend to occur one to four times per day over a period of several days. After one cluster of headaches is over, it may be months or even years before another occurs. Like migraines, cluster headaches are likely to be related to a dilation of the blood vessels in the brain, causing a localized increase in pressure.

The Economic Costs of Chronic Pain

Most people are surprised to learn that one in six Americans lives with chronic pain. While we might assume this condition is more prevalent among the elderly, a survey by Partners for Understanding Pain found that 80 percent of those with chronic pain are between 24 and 64 years of age. We might also tend to think of pain as a symptom of something else and not a condition in itself, but in fact, pain is the number one cause of disability in America. Chronic pain conditions cost an estimated $120 billion a year in medical costs and lost productivity. All those aches add up to a serious public health problem![8]

Personal Impact

If you're a person with chronic pain, every moment of your life is affected by it. Pain spills over into every aspect of life and can become your identity. It can make people lose everything, even their homes and their families. Unrelieved pain can lead to many consequences, such as depression, feelings of hopelessness, suicidal thoughts, increased stress, delayed

Did You Know?

- *80 percent of chronic pain sufferers are between the ages of 24 and 64.*
- *Over 75 million Americans are totally or partially disabled by serious pain, and more than 50 million suffer from chronic nonmalignant pain.*
- *Back pain, migraines, and arthritis alone account for actual medical costs of $40 billion annually.*

(Source: American Academy of Pain Medicine and American Pain Society.[8])

healing, hormonal imbalances, an impaired immune system, loss of appetite, insomnia, and needless suffering.

In fact, a recent survey found that 50 percent of chronic pain patients had considered suicide to escape the unrelenting agony of their pain. Requests for physician-assisted suicide are another indicator of pain's harsh impact on the quality of life for many patients and their families.

Current Treatments

Currently, the most common forms of medical treatment for chronic pain rely upon the use of powerful analgesic medications (painkillers), anti-inflammatories, and steroids, along with other medications to help manage the side effects of such strong drugs. While these medications may seem to be the miracle that allows pain sufferers to function, they are not actually solving the problem, just masking it. Medications may dull the symptoms, but they cannot cure the problem of chronic pain. As with all other physical problems, it is impossible to medicate our way out of the epidemic of chronic pain. Once again, the true solution lies in wellness.

Our Personal Health Care Bill
(based on a family of four)

Heart Disease	*$5,520 / year*	*$460 / month*
Cancer	*$2,876 / year*	*$240 / month*
Diabetes	*$1,808 / year*	*$151 / month*
Chronic Pain	*$1,643 / year* ·	*$137 / month*

*(Calculated by taking the total health care cost of these diseases
and dividing it by the total population.)*

Lifestyle Solutions

Spinal Alignment

Spinal adjustments have been repeatedly shown to be the most effective care for neck and back pain and headaches. Major studies demonstrate that spinal adjustments are more effective, cheaper, and have better long-term outcomes than any other treatment. This makes sense because spinal adjustments serve to re-establish normal vertebral motion and position in the spine. All other treatments, such as muscle relaxants, pain-killers and bed rest, only serve to decrease the symptoms of the problem and do not correct the problem itself.

A report released in 2001 by researchers at the Duke University Evidence-Based Practice Center in Durham, North

Carolina, found that "spinal manipulation resulted in almost immediate improvement for those headaches that originate in the neck, and had significantly fewer side effects and longer-lasting relief of tension-type headaches than commonly prescribed medications." These findings support an earlier study published in the *Journal of Manipulative and Physiological Therapeutics* that found spinal manipulative therapy to be very effective for treating tension headaches. This study also found that those who stopped receiving care after four weeks continued to experience a sustained benefit, in contrast to those patients who received only pain medication and no spinal adjustment.

In 1999, Blue Cross/Blue Shield of Kansas presented a study of health care statistics of different types of treatment for low back pain. The results showed that spinal adjustments were more cost-effective than anesthesiology, neurosurgery, neurology, physical therapy, orthopedic reconstructive surgery, physical medicine and rehabilitation, and rheumatology. This study confirmed what many others have in the past—that patients suffering from back problems benefit most by going to get their spines aligned.

Exercise

Back muscles—like any other muscle in the body—require adequate exercise to maintain strength and tone. While muscles in the buttocks and thighs are used to walk or climb a flight of stairs, deep back muscles and abdominal muscles are usually left inactive and unconditioned. Unless the back and abdominal muscles are specifically exercised, they will become weak and leave the low back susceptible to injury and pain.

Believe it or not, sitting for long periods of time is very stressful for the low back. The problem is that when you sit, your pelvis rolls backward, causing your low back to flatten, your psoas muscles to tighten, and your abdominal muscles to become weak. Then when you stand back up again, your low back gets pulled forward by the tight psoas muscles. Weak abdominal muscles combined with the tight psoas muscles cause an increase in the curve of the low back, called a "hyperlordosis," or swayback.

People who are managing their health can participate in a variety of sports and exercise programs. Physical exercise can reduce joint pain and stiffness and can increase flexibility, muscle strength, and endurance. It also helps with weight reduction and contributes to an improved sense of well-being. Before starting any exercise program, people with arthritis should talk with their wellness doctor.

Exercises that doctors often recommend include:

• *Range-of-motion exercises (e.g., stretching, yoga, and Pilates) to help maintain normal joint movement, maintain or increase flexibility, and relieve stiffness.*

• *Strengthening exercises (e.g., weight lifting) to maintain or increase muscle strength. Strong muscles help support and protect joints affected by arthritis.*

• *Aerobic or endurance exercises (e.g., walking, bicycling)*
  to improve cardiovascular fitness, help control weight,
  and improve overall well-being. Studies show that aerobic
  exercise can also reduce inflammation in some joints.

Nutrition

Another important part of a treatment program for chronic pain is a well-balanced diet. Along with exercise, a well-balanced diet helps people manage their body weight, decrease inflammation, stimulate healing, and help the body stay healthy overall. Foods, just like anything else, have the ability to either stress your body or to help your body heal. Foods that tend to be stressful on the body include dairy, eggs, wheat, and corn, as well as anything with monosodium glutamate (MSG), nitrates, or nitrites (as are found in processed foods). Certain environmental toxins may also contribute to the overall physical stress on your body. It is important that you eat as many clean, organically-grown fresh foods as possible.

There are also certain common foods associated with the onset of migraines, which should be avoided by those who are susceptible to these painful headaches. Foods prepared with monosodium glutamate (MSG), for example, can trigger headaches: soy sauce, meat tenderizer, and a variety of packaged foods contain this supposed "flavor enhancer." Repeated exposure to nitrite compounds can result in a dull, pounding headache that may be accompanied by a flushed face. Nitrites, which dilate blood vessels, are found in hot dogs and other processed meats.

These foods, as well as other factors such as stress, odors, menstrual periods, exposure to household chemicals, even your mood, may trigger a migraine. Keeping a headache diary will help you better understand which factors affect your headache pattern.

Healthy Thinking

What you think and say to yourself impacts how you feel. Anger, depression, frustration, or anxiety commonly accompanies pain: these emotions are natural responses, but they often make a painful situation worse. Your thoughts and your emotions are intimately connected. Once you become aware of this connection, you can begin to influence your own state of being. Notice what you are thinking when you are in pain or feeling angry or depressed. Negative thoughts increase a sense of loss of control and compound feelings of helplessness. Try replacing negative thoughts with positive, hopeful ones and notice the difference. Immediately you will have regained some control over your own experience.

Learn how to identify and reframe your negative self-talk (thoughts) and beliefs. You can start by writing three positive statements about yourself. You will find more exercises later in this book for managing the way you think about pain. Learning new coping skills is essential for reducing negative reactions to chronic pain.

5

Stress

Modern life is full of pressure, frustration, and stress. Worrying about job security, being overworked, driving in rush-hour traffic, arguing with your spouse, even dealing with medical bills—all these create stress. According to a recent survey by the American Psychology Association, more than half of all Americans report being concerned about the level of stress in their everyday lives. Most people are feeling overscheduled, overextended, and overstressed. By far, the most commonly reported source of stress in people's lives is workplace stress.

A Northwestern National Life Insurance Company study found that one in four employees rank their jobs as the greatest source of stress in their lives. And according to Gallup, 80 percent of employees suffer from job stress, with nearly 40 percent reporting that they need help in managing their stress.

According to a Princeton Survey Research study, three-quarters of employees believe that there is more on-the-job stress than a generation ago.

Many studies suggest that stress is a contributing factor in the development of chronic and degenerative conditions, such as heart disease and diabetes. High stress levels at work also lead to job burnout, reduction in productivity, ill health, job dissatisfaction, absenteeism, and increased turnover.

How Stress Affects Your Body

When you experience stress, your pituitary gland responds by increasing the release of a hormone called adrenocorticotropic hormone (ACTH). When the pituitary gland sends out this burst of ACTH, it is like an alarm system going off deep inside your brain. This alarm tells your adrenal glands, situated atop your kidneys, to release a flood of stress hormones into your bloodstream, including cortisol and adrenaline. These stress hormones cause a whole series of physiological changes in your body which can increase your heart rate and blood pressure, shut down your digestive system, and alter your immune system. Once the perceived threat is gone, the levels of cortisol and adrenaline in your bloodstream decline, at which point your heart rate and blood pressure and all of your other body functions return to normal.

If stressful situations pile up one after another, your body has no chance to recover. The long-term continuous activation of the stress-response system can disrupt almost all of your body's processes. Here are the ways different systems of your body respond to stress:

- *Digestive system: Stomachache or diarrhea is very common when you're stressed. Stress hormones slow the release of stomach acid and the emptying of the stomach. The same hormones also stimulate the colon, which speeds the passage of its contents.*

- *Immune system: Chronic stress tends to dampen your immune system, making you more susceptible to colds and other infections. Typically, your immune system responds to infection by releasing several substances that cause inflammation. Chronic systemic inflammation contributes to the development of many degenerative diseases.*

- *Nervous system: Stress has been linked with depression, anxiety, panic attacks, and dementia. Over time, the chronic release of cortisol can cause damage to several structures in the brain. Excessive amounts of cortisol can also cause sleep disturbances and a loss of sex drive.*

- *Cardiovascular system: As mentioned earlier, stress causes an increase in both heart rate and blood pressure and increases the risk of heart attacks and strokes.*

Each person may react to a specific stressor differently. Some people are naturally laid-back about almost everything, while others react strongly at the slightest hint of stress. If you have had any of the following conditions, it may be a sign that you are suffering from stress:

- *Anxiety*
- *Back pain*
- *Constipation*
- *Depression*
- *Fatigue*
- *Weight gain or loss*

- *Insomnia*
- *Relationship problems*
- *Shortness of breath*
- *Stiff neck*
- *Upset stomach*
- *Diarrhea*

The Economic Costs of Stress

Job stress costs American businesses hundreds of billions of dollars a year in employee burnout, turnover, higher absenteeism, lower production, and increased health care costs. The American Psychological Association estimates that 60 percent of all absences are due to stress-related issues, costing US companies more than $57 billion a year. Workers reporting themselves as "stressed" incur health care costs that are 46 percent higher, or $600 more per person, than other employees. American businesses spend more than $26 billion each year in disability payments and medical bills for stress-related conditions.[1-2]

The Health Effects of Work Stress

- *Twice the rate of heart and cardiovascular problems*
- *Two to three times the rate of anxiety, depression and demoralization*
- *Twice the rate of substance abuse*
- *Two to three times the rate of infectious diseases*
- *Five times the rate of certain cancers*
- *Three times the rate of back pain*
- *Two to three times the rate of interpersonal conflicts*
- *Two to three times the rate of injuries*

(Source: Lluminari® Landmark Study.)

It is little wonder, then, that the rising cost of health insurance has become the single biggest expense facing many American businesses. According to the Kaiser Family Foundation's *2004 Annual Employer Health Benefits Survey*, employer-sponsored health insurance premiums increased an average of 11.2 percent in 2004—the fourth consecutive year of double-digit growth—and these premiums rose at a rate about five times that of inflation and workers' earnings. Cardiovascular disease, America's number one killer, affects 71 million Americans each year, and costs the nation nearly $400 billion in treatment and lost productivity—and that is only one of many conditions proven to be related to stress!

Did You Know?

- *Workplace stress costs the nation more than $300 billion each year in health care, missed work and stress reduction efforts.*
- *Stress is responsible for 19 percent of employee absenteeism and 40 percent of employee turnover.*
- *Stress is responsible for creating 60 percent of the cost of workplace accidents.*
- *Research shows that 60 to 90 percent of doctor visits are stress-related.*
- *A landmark 20-year study conducted by the University of London concluded that unmanaged reactions to stress were a more dangerous risk factor for cancer and heart disease than either cigarette smoking or high cholesterol foods.*
- *90 percent of all disease is caused or complicated by stress.*

(Source: American Institute of Stress and Chrysalis Performance Strategies.)

Personal Impact

Stress is a very expensive epidemic, because it not only leads to direct costs of its own but also aggravates just about every other form of illness. Like every other national expense,

Our Personal Health Care Bill
(based on a family of four)

Heart Disease	*$5,520 / year*	*$460 / month*
Cancer	*$2,876 / year*	*$240 / month*
Diabetes	*$1,808 / year*	*$151 / month*
Chronic Pain	*$1,643 / year*	*$137 / month*
Stress	*$ 780 / year*	*$ 65 / month*

*(Calculated by taking the total health care cost of these diseases
and dividing it by the total population.)*

the health care costs of stress have to come from our pockets, in the form of taxes, increased product costs, and health insurance premiums. Current estimates say that stress costs every person in America $195 per year, or $780 for a family of four. This does not even take into account the extra expense incurred by the effects of stress on other conditions, such as cancer, heart disease, obesity, and chronic pain. According to the *Journal of Occupational and Environmental Medicine*, health care expenditures are nearly 50 percent greater for workers reporting high levels of stress.

Stress not only affects your health and your pocketbook, but it seeps into every aspect of your life, slowly sapping the joy out of your day-to-day activities. In fact, stress—particularly financial stress—is one of the most common reasons why families split apart. It is also the leading cause of a whole host of psychological, emotional, and social ills, including violence, depression, and substance abuse.[1-2]

Current Treatments

Unlike most other diseases that affect Americans, there really isn't any routine medical treatment for stress. Some doctors will prescribe antidepressants, such as Zoloft® or Prozac®, while others will prescribe an anxiolytic medication, such as imipramine or Buspar®. Because stress is due to an emotional reaction to life events and is not a biochemical condition like diabetes, drugs have a limited ability to alleviate stress. The most effective way to help relieve stress is through lifestyle habits such as improved spinal alignment, exercise, breathing exercises, and coping strategies.

Lifestyle Solutions

After decades of research, it is clear that the negative effects associated with stress are real. Fortunately, many companies have been taking the lead in addressing the epidemic of stress by instituting workplace wellness programs that include a significant stress-reduction component. The most effective of these programs are the ones that integrate physical activity and nutritional programs alongside stress-management training.

Businesses that have instituted activity-based workplace wellness programs have enjoyed a $3.00-$5.00 return on every dollar invested in the form of decreased health care costs, decreased absenteeism, increased productivity, decreased employee turnover, and reduced insurance costs.

The Congressional Caucus on "Stress Prevention: Its Impact on Health and Medical Savings" found that "some of the leading conditions that cause the greatest health burden in this country—heart disease, stroke, cancer, and severe depression —are linked to stress and to a large extent are preventable." One study on the risk of heart disease found that employees who are involved in an activity-based stress-reduction program at work have only one-third of the heart-related conditions afflicting those who were not involved. In addition, one-time cardiac patients, by learning to manage stress, reduced their risk of having another heart attack or heart problem by 74 percent![4]

Although you may not always be able to avoid stressful situations, there are a number of things that you can do to reduce the effect stress has on your body.

Exercise

Exercise is a good way to deal with stress because it is a healthy way to relieve your pent-up energy and tension. It also helps you get in better shape, which makes you feel better overall. By getting physically active, you can decrease your levels of anxiety and stress, and elevate your moods. Numerous studies have shown that people who begin exercise programs, either at home or at work, demonstrate a marked improvement in their ability to concentrate, are able to sleep better, suffer from fewer illnesses, suffer from less pain, and report a much higher quality of life than those who do not exercise. This is even true of people who had not begun an exercise program until they were in their 40s, 50s, 60s or even 70s. So if you want to feel better and improve your quality of life, get active!

Spinal Alignment

One of the consequences of stress is a tendency to unconsciously tense up our muscles—especially in the upper back and shoulder region. This chronic tension, often coupled with poor posture, frequently causes the vertebrae of the spine to become misaligned. As you read in previous chapters, this misalignment causes irritation of the spinal nerves, and this irritation, in turn, often leads to more muscle tension. In this way, muscle tension becomes both the cause and the consequence of stress—all the while, the misalignments of the spine worsen. This vicious cycle will continue until the affected area of the spine is realigned. Unfortunately, there is no way to do this on your own; it requires the care of a spinal alignment specialist. Most people experience a noticeable improvement in their stress almost immediately after a spinal adjustment.

Nutritional Supplements

There are two types of nutritional supplements that can help with stress: those that help to reduce stress, and those that help the body better cope with the effects of stress. Supplements that help to reduce stress belong to a class of herbs that help the body relax. Herbs such as chamomile, skullcap, valerian, and lavender help to clear a hurried mind and calm intense emotions. People typically drink these herbs as teas.

Supplements to help the body better cope with the physical effects of stress are the B-vitamins and zinc. When you are under stress, your need for zinc and the B-vitamins goes up considerably. If you don't have enough of these, your health will suffer, which is why people often become sick when they are under a lot of stress. Taking a B-complex supplement along with zinc will help to protect your body from the negative effects of stress.

Healthy Thinking

Most stress is caused by two factors: dealing with change and feeling out of control of the events in our life. While we cannot always foresee the changes we will face in our lives, we can exert control over how we plan to meet each day: we can choose whether we shall act with purpose throughout our day or whether we shall simply react to what life throws at us. Being in a reactive mode is a very stressful place to be. External events seem to control your actions, rather than your actions determining the external events in your life.

Psychologists call this the "locus of control." Those with an external locus of control—in which the external world dictates their actions—are always in a state of anxiety and stress and frequently suffer from depression. Conversely, those with an internal locus of control, who act with purpose regardless of how chaotic their external environment is, experience a greater sense of peace and empowerment.

Most Americans have an external locus of control and, because our world is in a constant state of change, feel stressed much of the time. The simplest way to shift from the stressful external locus of control to a tranquil internal locus of control is to take charge of the events in your life.

An event, in this context, can be any activity you engage in: a phone call, dinner, a meeting, watching television. List all of the events that you participate in on a daily basis and decide which ones are genuinely important to you and which ones matter less. For example, is spending time with your child or partner more important than watching the depressing evening news?

Once you have your list, schedule your time to act on those things that have the highest value to you. This brings you to an internal locus of control. Too often, we focus on things that seem urgent at the expense of things that are truly important. The key here is to act with purpose and to avoid procrastination. Procrastination is the killer of dreams. When we procrastinate, our events control us, our stress level increases, and we don't feel good about ourselves.

Relaxation Techniques

There are a variety of ways to relax and there is no one way that is best for everyone. The most important point is to make relaxation a habit. Some people feel guilty about relaxing because they think they always have to be accomplishing something. Well, the good news is that relaxing is accomplishing something. It is giving your mind and body the opportunity to rest and rejuvenate, which are essential to a sense of health and well-being. There is more information about relaxation in chapter 12.

6

Obesity

Obesity in the United States has become the greatest health crisis of our time, affecting more Americans than any other condition, according to the US Centers for Disease Control (CDC). Obesity rates have increased by more than 60 percent among adults in the past ten years, affecting 60 million American adults, and will soon overtake smoking as the number one preventable cause of death and disease. Since 1980, obesity rates have doubled among children and tripled among adolescents. The World Health Organization projects that by 2025, 45 to 50 percent of all US adults and 30 percent of all US children will suffer from obesity.[3-5]

Obesity is a chronic condition of carrying excessive body fat that frequently results in a significant impairment of health and can drastically affect your self-image. Obesity is defined as having a Body Mass Index (BMI) of greater than 25—BMI is a calculation using your height and your body weight—and should be regarded like any other illness. As mentioned previously, obesity is a major contributor to many chronic diseases and health risks, including Type 2 diabetes, hypertension, heart disease, stroke, breast cancer, colon cancer, gallbladder disease, and arthritis—that's a huge strain on your body and on the total health care system!

In most cases, obesity is a lifestyle disease, primarily due to lack of activity and poor eating habits. It is true that some people have a genetic predisposition to weight gain; however, this is a very small percentage. For most of us, being overweight is simply a sign that we are not living optimally, in accordance with our physiological design: we need to turn our attention to what we eat and how much movement we create in our lives.

If you are overweight, you are certainly not alone. Many theories attempt to account for the rising rates of obesity: factors include sedentary lifestyles, excessive consumption, genetics, stress, and depression; even food additives can play a role. In most cases, obesity is the result of a combination of factors, so overcoming the problem will require dietary changes, increased activity levels, and new healthy thinking patterns.

First, let us examine ways in which obesity affects our health.

Hypertension

Hypertension is the medical name for high blood pressure. With the significant rise in obesity in the last decade, we have seen a corresponding increase in the incidence of hypertension.

Though not all people who are overweight also suffer from high blood pressure, studies indicate that approximately 75 percent of hypertension cases are directly attributable to excessive weight. This makes obesity the single greatest cause of hypertension in the American population.

Typically, obesity contributes to hypertension through what is referred to as "peripheral resistance," which simply means that it is harder for blood to flow through an overweight body. Peripheral resistance, combined with the fact that the heart has to pump extra blood to all of the extra tissue in the body, results in high blood pressure. High blood pressure increases your risk of a heart attack, stroke, kidney failure, and macular degeneration.

Studies have shown weight loss to be the most effective nonpharmacological therapy for lowering blood pressure in those who are overweight. There is a direct correlation between the degree of weight loss and the reduction in blood pressure. Even modest weight loss of five to ten percent of body weight yields clinically significant reductions in blood pressure.[6]

Type 2 Diabetes

This chronic elevation in blood sugar is a major cause of early death, heart disease, kidney disease, stroke, and blindness. Also, people who have diabetes or pre-diabetes are more likely to suffer fatty liver disease—a condition similar to alcoholic liver damage—whether or not they ever drink alcohol.

More than 80 percent of people with Type 2 diabetes are overweight. It may be that excessive weight causes cells to change, making them less effective at using sugar from the blood. More commonly, however, those who are obese develop insulin resistance, in which the tissues of the body lose their sensitivity to insulin.[2,7]

You can lower your risk for developing Type 2 diabetes by losing weight and increasing your amount of physical activity. If you have Type 2 diabetes, losing weight and becoming more physically active can help you control your blood sugar levels and, in some cases, actually reverse the disease. Weight loss, exercise, and nutritional supplements may also allow you to reduce your diabetes medication.

Coronary Artery Disease

The coronary arteries are the arteries that feed the heart. When they become clogged with cholesterol, the blood flow to the heart is restricted. This is known as coronary artery disease. People who are overweight are more likely to suffer from high levels of triglycerides (blood fats), elevated LDL cholesterol (a fat-like substance often called "bad cholesterol"), and insufficient HDL cholesterol (often called "good cholesterol"). These are all risk factors for coronary artery disease and stroke. In addition, people with more body fat have higher blood levels of substances that cause inflammation—this further raises the risk of heart disease.

Even losing five to ten percent of your body weight can significantly lower your chances of developing heart disease or having a stroke. If you weigh 200 pounds, this means losing as little as ten pounds.[8]

Gallbladder Disease

People who are overweight have a higher risk of developing gallbladder disease and gallstones. Gallstones are clusters, mostly of cholesterol, that form in the gallbladder and can cause severe abdominal or back pain.

Weight loss that is too rapid—three or more pounds per week—can actually increase your chance of developing gallstones. Modest, slow weight loss of about one-half to two pounds per week is a much healthier alternative and will not increase your risk of developing gallstones.

Cancer

Being overweight increases your risk of developing several types of cancer, including cancers of the colon, esophagus, and kidney, as well as uterine and postmenopausal breast cancer in women. Once cancer occurs, obesity increases the likelihood of patient fatality. The exact correlation between excessive body weight and cancer growth is not known, but the current thinking is that fat cells make hormones that can affect cell growth, and these abnormally high hormone levels ultimately lead to cancer.

Several studies have shown that losing weight can dramatically reduce the cancer risk in people who are overweight.

Metabolic Syndrome

A metabolic syndrome is a cluster of medical conditions characterized by insulin resistance, the presence of obesity, abdominal fat, high blood sugar, elevated triglycerides, high blood cholesterol, and high blood pressure. In 2002, the *Journal of the American Medical Association* reported that as many as forty-seven million Americans may exhibit a metabolic syndrome. The root causes of this condition are typically poor diet and insufficient physical activity. Currently, the most effective way to avoid or overcome metabolic syndrome is through a comprehensive program of diet and exercise.

Overall Quality of Life

Along with increasing your risk of disease, obesity also saps your energy and damages your quality of life. Obesity carries a large social stigma: people who are overweight frequently struggle with poor body image, low self-esteem, and depression. Obesity may limit social mobility. It may even disrupt the normal hormonal pathways.

There is a chemical link between obesity and stress: it is centered in the hormonal pathway known as the HPA axis, the route of communication between the hypothalamus (the peanut-

Did You Know?

The direct medical costs for diseases related to obesity are approximately:

- *$98 billion per year for Type 2 diabetes*
- *$8.8 billion per year for heart disease*
- *$5.3 billion per year for osteoarthritis*
- *$3.2 billion per year for gallbladder disease*
- *$1.3 billion for colon cancer*
- *$1.1 billion for breast cancer*
- *$310 million for endometrial cancer*

(Source: The US Centers for Disease Control.)

sized part of the brain that governs parts of the nervous system), the pituitary gland, and the adrenal glands. These three points of the body work together to maintain chemical equilibrium when the body is under stress.

The HPA axis is responsible for releasing cortisol, the so-called stress hormone, which plays a critical role in energy metabolism, as well as other functions. The problem with cortisol is that it prompts the body to deposit fat around the abdomen: this pattern of fat storage is especially hazardous to health.

The Economic Costs of Obesity

In 2003, the total health care cost due to obesity in the United States was estimated at $137 billion, of which $75 billion went towards direct medical costs and $62 billion to indirect costs.[9-10] This means an expense of approximately $257 per year for every single American.

The cost in death, disability, and lost productivity from obesity has come close to that of tobacco. A recent report notes that tobacco use is responsible for approximately 440,000 deaths per year, whereas obesity is responsible for at least 300,000 deaths per year. Those who are obese suffer 30 to 50 percent more health problems than smokers or problem drinkers.[11]

The lifetime medical costs of the five major diseases related to obesity—hypertension, diabetes, heart disease, stroke, and high cholesterol—are $10,000 higher among moderately obese people than among those who maintain a healthy weight. A ten percent weight loss will reduce an overweight person's lifetime medical costs by $2,200-$5,300.[12]

Personal Impact

As with the other conditions discussed earlier, each one of us is responsible for paying the bill for the health costs associated with obesity. Taxpayers foot the doctor's bill for more than half of obesity-related medical costs through the Medicare and

Our Personal Health Care Bill
(based on a family of four)

Heart Disease	*$5,520 / year*	*$460 / month*
Cancer	*$2,876 / year*	*$240 / month*
Diabetes	*$1,808 / year*	*$151 / month*
Chronic Pain	*$1,643 / year*	*$137 / month*
Stress	*$ 780 / year*	*$ 65 / month*
Obesity	*$1,027 / year*	*$ 86 / month*

*(Calculated by taking the total health care cost of these diseases
and dividing it by the total population.)*

Medicaid programs, which run $75 billion per year in direct medical costs, or about $175 per person. This doesn't even take into account the increased health insurance premiums paid and the higher prices paid at the cash register to cover the remaining expenses.[9-10]

While the financial costs associated with obesity are quite dramatic, there is a human cost, as well. People who are overweight tend to suffer from depression, low self-esteem, and stress. This is due in part to the constant bombardment of size-obsessed media images; but it is also a matter of chemistry. As people become more overweight, changes in brain chemistry and hormone levels can disrupt their psychological well-being.

Current Medical Treatments

Currently, the primary medical option for treating obesity is a surgical procedure called the "gastric bypass," which is the term for any surgery intended to alter the digestive process in an effort to help someone lose weight. Gastric bypass operations can be divided into three types: restrictive, malabsorptive, and combined restrictive/malabsorptive.

Restrictive operations limit food intake by creating a narrow passage from the upper part of the stomach into the larger lower part, reducing the amount of food the stomach can hold and slowing the passage of food through the stomach. Malabsorptive operations do not limit food intake, but instead exclude most of the small intestine from the digestive tract so fewer calories and nutrients are absorbed. Malabsorptive operations, also called intestinal bypasses, are no longer recommended because they result in severe nutritional deficiencies. Combined operations use stomach restriction and a partial bypass of the small intestine.

Each of these procedures is both physically drastic and expensive, and none of them addresses the underlying causes of obesity. The country's and the individual's health care dollars could be more effectively spent on prevention care and lifestyle modifications. If we regard obesity as a disease, then once again we need to do what we can to have more people who are less sick!

Lifestyle Solutions

Weight Loss Programs

According to a report from the Institute of Medicine (IOM) entitled *Weighing The Options: Criteria for Evaluating Weight Management Programs*, tens of millions of Americans are dieting at any given time and spending more than $33 billion yearly on weight-reduction products or diet foods and drinks. Yet, studies over the last two decades by the National Center for Health Statistics show that the number of Americans who are overweight is actually on the rise.

The fact is that many people who diet fail to lose weight, or if they do lose weight, they fail to maintain the lower weight over the long term. Fad diets or pills that promise a quick and easy path to thinness usually deliver only disappointment in the end. Lasting, healthy weight loss is only achievable through a comprehensive lifestyle program.

Because many factors affect a person's body weight, such as how much or how little food a person eats, how the food is metabolized by the body, and how much daily activity a person gets, losing weight is not as simple as eating less. Maintaining a healthy body weight requires a change in lifestyle that includes dietary changes, an increase in activity level, healthy spinal alignment, stress reduction, and a positive mental attitude.

Exercise

You do not have to be an athlete to benefit from regular physical activity. Even modest amounts of physical activity can improve your health. Start with small, specific goals such as walking ten minutes a day, three days a week, and slowly build up from there. Keep an activity log to track your progress. Try these activities to add more movement to your daily life:

- *Take the stairs instead of the elevator.*
- *Get off the bus one stop early if you are in an area safe for walking.*
- *Park the car farther away from entrances to stores, movie theaters, or your home.*
- *Take a short walk around the block with family, friends, or co-workers.*
- *In bad weather, walk around a mall.*
- *Rake the leaves or wash the car.*
- *Visit museums, the zoo, or an aquarium. You and your family can walk for hours and not realize it.*
- *Take a walk after dinner instead of watching television.*

As you become more fit, slowly increase your pace, the length of time you are active, and how often you are active. If you are a man over age 40 or a woman over age 50, or if you have chronic health problems, check with your health care provider before beginning a program of vigorous activity.

For a well-rounded workout plan, combine aerobic activity, muscle-strengthening exercises, and stretching. Do at least 30 minutes a day of moderate physical activity on most or all days of the week. Add muscle-strengthening activities to your aerobic workout two to three times a week.

To reduce the risk of injury, do a slow warm-up and then stretch before aerobic or strengthening activities. Follow your workout with a few more minutes of stretching.

Aerobic activity is any activity that speeds up your heart and breathing while moving your body. If you have been inactive for a while, you may want to start with easier activities, such as walking at a gentle pace. You can then build up to more intense activity without hurting your body. Here are some of the health advantages of regular aerobic activity:

- *Control weight: Aerobic activity burns calories, which may help you manage your weight.*
- *Prevent heart disease and stroke: Regular aerobic activity can strengthen your heart muscle and lower your blood pressure. It may also help lower cholesterol.*
- *Maintain strong bones: Weight-bearing aerobic activities that involve lifting or pushing your own body weight— such as walking, jogging, or dancing—help to maintain strong bones.*
- *Improve your outlook: Aerobic exercise relieves tension and decreases stress. As you get fit, your confidence and self-image will improve.*

Start an activity log to record your minutes of activity each day. Choose aerobic activities that are fun. People are more likely to be active if they like what they are doing. It also helps to get support from a friend or a family member. Try one of these activities, or others you enjoy:

- *Brisk walking or jogging*
- *Bicycling*
- *Swimming*
- *Aerobic exercise classes*
- *Dancing (square dancing, salsa, African dance, swing)*
- *Playing basketball or soccer*

Strengthening activities include lifting weights, using resistance bands, and doing push-ups or sit-ups. Besides building stronger muscles, strengthening activities may help you to:

- *Use more calories: Not only does the exercise burn calories, but having more muscle means you will burn more calories—even when you are sitting still.*
- *Reduce injury: Stronger muscles improve balance and support your joints, reducing the risk of injury.*
- *Maintain strong bones: Doing strengthening exercises regularly helps build bone and may prevent bone loss as you age.*

Strengthening exercises should focus on working the major muscle groups of the body, such as the chest, back, and legs. Do exercises for each muscle group two or three times a week. Allow at least one day of rest for your muscles to recover and rebuild before another strengthening workout.

Exercise Tips for the Very Large

Very large people face special challenges in trying to be active. You may not be able to bend or move in the same way that other people can. It may be hard to find clothes and equipment for exercising, and you may feel self-conscious being physically active around other people. Facing these challenges is hard, but it can be done!

When starting your exercise program, it is important to be easy on yourself. If you cannot do an activity, don't feel bad about it. Just feel good about what you can do and avoid negative self-talk. One very heavy woman once said that if other people talked to her the way she sometimes talks to herself, she would punch them. Focus on the positive and you will improve your chances of success.

If you are a large person starting on an exercise program, it is important to start slowly. Your body needs time to get used to your new activity. Be sure to spend some time warming up. Warm-ups get your body ready for action. Shrug your shoulders, tap your toes, swing your arms, or march in place. You should spend a few minutes warming up for any physical activity, even walking. Move more slowly for the first few minutes. Spend some time cooling down. Slow down little by little. If you have been walking fast, walk slowly or stretch for a few minutes to cool down. Cooling down protects your heart, relaxes your muscles, and keeps you from getting hurt.

Be sure to pay attention to your body. If you are very large, your joints will be supporting much more weight. If your feet, knees, or back begin to hurt from weight-bearing exercise, start out by doing non-weight-bearing exercise and slowly work up to doing weight-bearing exercise. Listening to your body will help you avoid potential injuries that could set you back.

If you are not active now, start slowly. Try to walk just four minutes per day for the first week. Walk eight minutes per day the next week. Stay at eight minute walks until you feel comfortable. Then increase your walks to twelve minutes. Slowly lengthen each walk by four minutes per week until you reach 20 minutes per day. Once you reach 20 minutes per day, you can work on quickening your pace to get your walking into the aerobic range. Please be patient! You will be much better off in the long run if you start slowly and build up endurance.

7

Drug Reactions

According to *The New England Journal of Medicine*, the percentage of the personal health care dollars spent on prescription drugs has grown faster than any other segment, including doctor and hospital bills. America has a mania for medication, but in a growing number of cases, these drugs do more harm than good.

Each year approximately 2.2 million US hospital patients experience adverse drug reactions (ADRs) from taking prescription medications. Of these, 106,000 patients die.[1] Because the safety of a new drug cannot be known with certainty until it has been on the market for many years, even FDA-approved drugs can be the source of serious ADRs.[10] Three to six percent of all hospital admissions are the result of adverse drug reactions, and six to fifteen percent of hospitalized patients experience a serious adverse drug reaction.[8-11] The economic cost of ADRs is more than $12 billion per year.[2-5]

Pharmaceutical Marketing and Lobbying

More than a third of pharmaceutical companies' resources go into promotion and marketing. Annually, the industry spends up to $60 billion on drug marketing—nearly twice what it spends on research and development. In an effort to promote prescription drugs to the widest audience possible, drug companies run advertisements directly to consumers. In 2004, Pfizer spent almost $120 million for media ads for Lipitor®, the

Pharmaceutical Spending on Marketing

Company	Marketing	Research
Pfizer	*$16.90 billion*	*$7.68 billion*
GlaxoSmithKline	*$12.93 billion*	*$5.20 billion*
Sanofi-Aventis	*$5.59 billion*	*$9.26 billion*
Johnson & Johnson	*$15.86 billion*	*$5.20 billion*
Merck	*$7.35 billion*	*$4.01 billion*
Novartis	*$8.87 billion*	*$4.21 billion*
AstraZeneca	*$7.84 billion*	*$3.80 billion*
Hoffman La Roche	*$7.24 billion*	*$4.01 billion*
Bristol-Myers Squibb	*$6.43 billion*	*$2.50 billion*
Wyeth	*$5.80 billion*	*$2.46 billion*
Abbott Labs	*$4.92 billion*	*$1.70 billion*

(Source: The Center for Public Integrity.[17])

world's number-one selling prescription drug, while companies promoting the erectile dysfunction treatments Viagra®, Levitra®, and Cialis® spent $425 million. Direct-to-consumer advertising has also grown significantly: from $791 million in 1996 to $3.8 billion in 2004.[6-7] And that represents only 15 percent of the total pharmaceutical advertising budget! Where does that money come from? You guessed it—your pocket!

While the drug companies maintain that direct-to-consumer advertising is educational, Dr. Sidney M. Wolfe of the Public Citizen Health Research Group in Washington, D.C., argues that the public often is misinformed about these ads: viewers mistakenly believe that "the FDA reviews all ads before they are released and allows only the safest and most effective drugs to be promoted directly to the public." This is simply not the case.

People want what they see on television. They are told to go to their doctors for a prescription. Doctors in private practice either acquiesce to their patients' demands for these drugs or spend valuable time trying to talk patients out of medications which are inappropriate or unnecessary.[8-9]

The pharmaceutical and health products industry has also spent more than $800 million for lobbying efforts at the federal and state levels over the past seven years, more than any other industry group, except the insurance industry.[10] These efforts have defeated several measures aimed at containing drug prices. They have blocked the importation of medicines from countries that cap prescription drug prices. The drug industry's huge investments in Washington have produced a series of favorable laws on Capitol Hill and resulted in tens of billions of dollars in additional profits.

Take for example Medicare Part D: to date, around 90 percent of those eligible for Medicare Part D have enrolled in the drug plan, and large pharmaceutical companies and insurers are reporting huge increases in their profits. In early August 2006, the *Wall Street Journal* reported a 4.9 percent increase in prescription drug sales and as much as a 20 percent increase in drug companies' profits, all attributable to Medicare Part

---

Did You Know?

- *HMOs spend more treating ADRs than on drugs.[18]*
- *ADRs are the cost leader for malpractice payouts.[18]*
- *Up to one-third of drug prescriptions are not needed and therefore wasted.*
- *The Government Accounting Office (GAO) reports that 51 percent of new drugs have serious, undetected adverse effects at the time of approval.*
- *Of the best selling prescription drugs, 148 can cause depression, 133 hallucinations or psychoses, 105 constipation, 76 dementia, 27 insomnia, and 36 Parkinsonism.[19]*

(Source: The Food and Drug Administration,[7] J Am Pharm Assoc 41:192.[18-19])

D. At the same time, private insurers, such as WellPoint, Inc. (the nation's largest insurer, with a reported enrollment of 1.5 million people in its Medicare plans), are enjoying huge profit gains.

Personal Impact

The overuse of prescription drugs indicates the level of our country's health crisis but does not offer any solution. Medication does not address the leading causes of disease: (a) spinal stress and its adverse affects on the immune system and

Our Personal Health Care Bill
(based on a family of four)

Heart Disease	*$5,520 / year*	*$460 / month*
Cancer	*$2,876 / year*	*$240 / month*
Diabetes	*$1,808 / year*	*$151 / month*
Chronic Pain	*$1,643 / year*	*$137 / month*
Stress	*$ 780 / year*	*$ 65 / month*
Obesity	*$1,027 / year*	*$ 86 / month*
Drug Reactions	*$ 164 / year*	*$ 14 / month*
Total Bill:	***$13,818 / year***	***$1,152 / month***

(Calculated by taking the total health care cost of these diseases and dividing it by the total population.)

nervous system; (b) insufficient exercise; (c) excessive caloric intake; (d) chronic mental and emotional stress; and (e) making unhealthy lifestyle choices.

The incredible cost associated with adverse drug reactions and excessive drug use drives home the point that we cannot medicate our way to health. Once again, the answer is to have more people less sick! This has been said over and over again, because it is the central message of this book. Health care, as it is conducted today, can never lead to a healthier population because it does not promote the fundamental secret to health: wellness.

Wellness is not found in a pill, a hospital, or under the surgeon's knife. In fact, these things are only indications of an unhealthy lifestyle. Wellness is found in the way you think about yourself and the world around you. If you truly want to become rich in every sense of the word, it is crucial to adopt a way of life that will create well-being.

SPECIAL SECTION

Perspectives on Wellness

By Dr. Michael Zimmerman, M.D.
Family Physician

I would like to offer some important context for the fine work Dr. Bob Hoffman and Dr. Jason A. Deitch have put forth in this book. Their clear intent is to offer us a prescription for re-empowerment. Perhaps the most startling aspect of this book is that it does not teach us ideas we do not already know. Rather, through the process we are reacquainted with our natural, innate intuition about our own health and "wellness." This journey is about restoring and realigning the confidence and control that we have lost in our health and lives. For some, *Discover Wellness* will take them back to a place that is cozy and familiar, offering a rediscovery of health and wellness that had been previously known but long lost. For others, the journey may offer a new center, one never before experienced.

Before we move on with the journey we should ask ourselves just how did we get so lost, so detached, so off-center to need such a guide to reacquaint ourselves with ourselves? There are multiple reasons for this detachment, I feel. As a practicing family physician and an active participant in efforts to improve health care in America, I wonder about the contribution of our "health care" system itself. Perhaps Dr. Hoffman's and Dr. Deitch's message has something to offer the wayward American health care system as well as the individual.

Generally, the American health care experience is one in which things are done to you rather than with you. In this process you quickly become disconnected from the "real" you. This detachment is seen at many levels. Insurance restrictions, poor office management, or "busy" medical staff can limit your access to care, information, and services. Delays are the rule and the expectation is that you will wait. Do you know any other business that has a "waiting room," or at least has the nerve to call it that? At times you are literally depersonalized as you are given an arm tag, undressed, and issued a standardized gown. Unbeknownst to you, your name has even been changed, perhaps you are "the 10:20 appointment" or the "hyper-tensive, arthritic in room 342." Most interactions are a set-up for your minimization. The doctor is standing, you are sitting. The doctor is dressed in a coat of authority and you are lucky to be only half-naked. You are generally outside this process, and if you should enter into it, you are treated as an object within it.

Clearly this experience does little to promote patient engagement in management of disease, let alone in one's own health and wellness. In fact, the result is often quite the opposite. It is critical to understand that this is not about bad people. Providers at all levels of the health care system are tremendously hard working, passionate and caring. In fact, the experience from within the health care system is equally frustrating.

Like most of my colleagues, I chose to take the rigorous path of becoming a family physician because I wanted to positively impact the lives of people in need. I like to help people, and I find that in the right environment, I am quite good at it, as many physicians are. We make tremendous sacrifices to become doctors. Unless you know someone who has done it, you cannot imagine the amount of effort, studying, personal investment, and time away from your family involved in becoming a doctor. It is tremendous. I love being a doctor because I love being able to save lives and truly help people who are in need.

I can give you this perspective from my actual experience as a family physician who is on the front lines of medicine, who delivers babies in the middle of the night, who rushes to the hospital because of someone's asthma attack, and who daily listens to people's fears about how sick they are: today's health care system does not allow doctors to deliver the best of medicine.

I would like to demonstrate how the experience one has within the health care system is largely a product of the model upon which it operates. In the present model, the health care of the patient is seen to occur in one of three major areas. The most basic is Primary Care: this would traditionally include interactions with your family doctor, pediatrician, or internist in the office setting. Secondary Care is the domain of the specialist such as the cardiologist or orthopedist and may include services at your local community hospital. Tertiary Care is delivered by the super subspecialist such as the liver transplant surgeon, usually at an academic medical center. The patient is an object that passes through and around this system. The focus of the system is to fit you into its "boundaries." Little, if any, attention is given to anything outside.

I would suggest that the fatal flaw in this view and a large component of the present failure of American health care is that it neglects to account for and integrate the arena where the great majority of true "health care" actually takes place: that is, patient self-care, family care, and community care. I would argue that this model is one key factor that further disconnects the individual, family, and community from their natural, innate connection with health and wellness. Instead of participating in a process to help heal disease, a person becomes a "patient," seeking a diagnosis in order to receive treatment from the proper specialist. Instead of promoting and facilitating health care at home, at work, and in your community, we fail to provide either the "health" or the "care" that is the premise of the model. Ironically, the present system in which I practice hinders the capability of hard-working providers to deliver truly optimal clinical outcomes and, I would argue, adds significant expense.

Clearly, one of the central failures of America's health care system is its disregard and underestimation of a person while she or he is "outside" the "boundaries" of the system. In this context it is certainly not a surprise to find that health care in America is incredibly expensive, wasteful, inefficient, and prone to error. We have been trying to run a health care system while ignoring where the majority of health care takes place!

A more enlightened view sees the present health care model as just the tip of the iceberg. When we look below the surface we find that the majority of health care, whether wellness or disease management, occurs outside our antiquated definitions of the domain of health care.

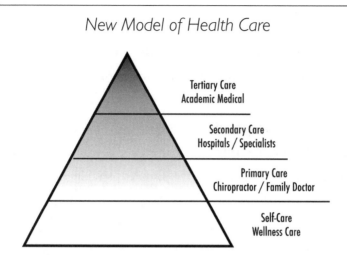

New Model of Health Care

Tertiary Care
Academic Medical

Secondary Care
Hospitals / Specialists

Primary Care
Chiropractor / Family Doctor

Self-Care
Wellness Care

Acknowledging that the person, family, and community are the locations of the majority of actual care will be fundamental to the successful reengineering of America's health care system. Furthermore, we must understand that people themselves are not only the center of a new quality health care system but, in fact, are ready, willing, and able to be the lead providers of health care for themselves, their families, and for their communities.

Where the old model further served to alienate individuals from themselves, the focus of the new model commits the health care system to actively engage and assist people, their families, and communities into taking responsibility for their own health, wellness, and disease management. This perspective is a tremendous shift and will have profound implications in policy and practice.

Rather than being a burden on this new health care system, the incorporation of self-care and personal responsibility offers a rich and bountiful previously untapped resource.

I write this to you as someone who is in the present health care system every single day. I am not an insurance executive, pharmaceutical industry spokesman, or hospital administrator. I am a medical doctor taking care of people just like you everyday. I can tell you that health care in the United States is in a time of great flux. The present system is in shambles. Costs are astronomical and quality of care is unacceptably poor. The reengineering of health care in America is a monumentally complex task. Like many of us, health care in America has lost its center; it has become out of touch with its true purpose and goals. It will require vision and fundamental transformation.

As I read through *Discover Wellness*, I wonder if there are lessons to help all of us in the transformation of America's health care system. I wonder if the prescription for realignment and refocusing for people just like you and me isn't also applicable to the health care system itself.

It is my hope as a family physician, along with the hundreds of thousands of others doctors like me, that we have the foresight to see the dangers our present system faces, the intelligence to make good decisions, and the courage to make the changes necessary to create a new and better way of thinking about and experiencing our innate health and wellness. As a family physician and concerned citizen, I encourage you to take an active role in your own health. I have hopes that America's health care system is able to rediscover that you, your family, and your community are where health care happens. I encourage you to *Discover Wellness*.

8

Discover Wellness

We are witnessing a significant shift away from conventional medicine and towards an ongoing wellness lifestyle. The "outside-in" allopathic model of disease-care is being superseded by the "inside-out" wellness model of health care. At the same time, we see our country transitioning from a manufacturing-driven economy to an idea-driven economy. These changes are not unrelated. It is increasingly clear that Americans have made the decision to take greater responsibility for their health and their quality of life.

Some have called this trend "the human potential movement," and others refer to it as "the wellness revolution." Whatever you choose to call it, the premise is based on having a profound respect for the body's ability to heal itself; people have been teaching this core principle of wellness for thousands of years. Now, in our idea-driven economy, wellness is an idea whose time has returned.

Traditional "health care" is really a sickness business: it only functions reactively, after people have become sick. Enormous sums are spent treating existing disease: according to Paul Zane Pilzer, a leading economist and author, approximately one-seventh of the United States economy, or about $1.8 trillion, is devoted to this sickness business, what we erroneously call "health care." But now the idea of wellness, of focusing health care on staying healthy, is gaining prevalence. The significant shift away from conventional medicine and towards the wellness model of health care has been and continues to be fueled by the information revolution and by the aging Baby Boomer generation. According to journalist Anna Quindlen, the greatest advance in health care in our lifetime has not been transplants or new pharmaceuticals: it has been the rise of the informed consumer.

In the past, people who chose to breast feed, exercise daily, meditate, take vitamins, and/or go to the chiropractor on a regular basis would be scoffed at for being "health nuts." Today, it is the people who do not participate in these types of activities who are considered to be out of step. Yes, Americans are increasingly obsessed with health and with maximizing their quality of life.

Moving Away from Medications

We are learning and relearning daily that the old maxim "better health through better chemistry" is not a solution.

Examples of conventional medicine's failure abound in the press. One study by researchers at the University of Texas Southwestern Medical Center tracked more than 300 cases of acute liver failure at 22 hospitals and found that 38 percent of the liver failures were associated with excessive acetaminophen use. What is considered excessive? According to the *New England Journal of Medicine*, excessive use is defined as "taking more than 1,000 pills in a lifetime, or more than 365 pills in a year." The people who dose themselves daily with these over-the-counter "pain killers" find their medicine has been killing them.

Every day in North America, millions of children diagnosed as suffering from attention deficit disorder (ADD) or attention deficit hyperactivity disorder (ADHD) are chemically "lobotomized." Yet more than 30 years ago, the World Health Organization classified methylphenidate (Ritalin®), one of the most popular pharmaceutical "solutions" to these conditions, as a Schedule 2 drug—the same class as cocaine and PCP—because of its highly addictive qualities and high potential for abuse. Should we, as Americans, be okay with this? Should our children be put on medications like this with little research into their long-term effects?

The American Medical Association has estimated that 40 to 60 percent of the more than 2 billion prescriptions written by doctors each year are provided "off-label": this means that the drugs prescribed are not tested or FDA-approved for treating the condition they are being prescribed for. Dr. Richard Greene, the director for the Agency for Health Care Policy and Research, has said, "The public is shocked when they learn that there isn't a shred of evidence for a lot of medical therapies. They just can't believe their doctors are doing things they can't back up."

"You need to know that the current health care system is designed to create fear," according to Dr. Joe Mercola. We need to become better educated about the dangers of medicine and the benefits of wellness. Dr. Mercola, the founder of Mercola.com, is a pioneer of using the Internet to bring natural health and wellness information to the public. Mercola.com has become the world's most visited natural health Web site in the world with almost one million subscribers and over five million page views every month. "Over 80 percent of the people on the Internet search health information, but unfortunately there is as yet no destination spot for health information—and the field is loaded with fraud and deception," says Dr. Mercola. His newest Web site, VitalVotes.com, is a treasure trove of knowledge and health wisdom. We all need more resources to help us learn what most of the media is not yet reporting on: how to have better health through better living.

Better Health through Better Living Is the Answer

So, if better health through better chemistry has failed, what other options exist? Millions of Americans are discovering and adopting a new health care paradigm, which is "better health through better living." What was once considered "alternative medicine" has become increasingly accepted into the mainstream: it continues to grow into the preferred form of true health care.

In the United States, 36 percent of adults use some form of "Complementary Alternative Medicine" (CAM), according to national study results released in 2004 by the National Center for Complementary and Alternative Medicine (NCCAM), a division of the National Institutes of Health (NIH). When megavitamin therapy and prayer specifically for health reasons are included in the definition of CAM, that number rises to 62 percentage. The study also included a survey to discover why people use CAM. Here we see a sample of the responses:

- *55 percent of adults said they were most likely to use CAM because they believed that it would help them when combined with conventional medical treatments.*
- *50 percent thought that CAM would be interesting to try.*
- *26 percent used CAM because a conventional medical professional suggested that they try it.*
- *13 percent used CAM because they felt that conventional medicine was too expensive.*

The survey also found that approximately 28 percent of adults used CAM because they believed conventional medical treatments would not help them with their health problems.

As reported in *The Trends Journal* a few years ago, "A growing number of prominent doctors are bucking establishment dogma. They allege that physicians, once seen as approaching the divine, can't help 80 percent of disease. They also say that medicine and surgery only cure ten percent of disease and that at least another ten percent of diseases are caused by accidents of surgery and side-effects of medicine."

Prominent physicians who have successfully shifted to a more natural and body-respectful focus on wellness care include Dr. Andrew Weil, Dr. Dean Ornish, Dr. Julian Whitaker, and Dr. Deepak Chopra, to name just a few. One of the most powerful statements on this health model comes from Dr. Chopra: "Inside your body is a wonderful pharmacy. You name it, and the human body can make it... tranquilizers, sleeping pills, anti-cancer drugs; the right dose at the right time for the right organ with no side effects. And all the instructions you need come with the packaging, which is your innate intelligence."

What Is Wellness?

Wellness can be defined as the quality or state of being healthy; especially as the result of deliberate effort, or as an approach to health care that emphasizes preventing illness and prolonging life, as opposed to emphasizing the treatment of diseases. Additionally, Dr. Patrick Gentempo, CEO of Creating Wellness, defines wellness as the degree to which an individual experiences health and vitality in any dimension of life.

Wellness requires you to be a proactive agent for your body. You need to treat it well and not wait until you hurt before you decide to take care of it. As I've said before, health is not merely the absence of disease any more than wealth is an absence of poverty. Let's remember health is not simply "feeling fine," for we know that problems may progress for years without causing any symptoms whatsoever. As you know by now, heart disease, for example, often develops unnoticed for many years before it strikes: in fact, the first symptom of heart disease that many people experience is a heart attack or death.

Now let us be clear that I am not under the illusion that everyone who creates a wellness lifestyle will be immune from pain, sickness, and disease. There are many people who do everything right and still get sick and die. Some will argue that there are many people who do everything wrong and live long, seemingly healthy lives. However, since we have no way to predict who is who, we have to do our very best to reduce our risk and promote our health.

Over the years in private practice, I have seen how neglecting their health has drained people of thousands of dollars, sometimes to the point of bankruptcy. I have seen people who have saved up and waited their entire lives to take a dream trip or to send their kids to college, whose savings and dreams were siphoned away to pay for health care expenses. I have seen people with work injuries like carpal tunnel syndrome or neck and back pain who have been unable to work, unable to drive, and even unable to sleep without pain. I have seen family members whose entire lives become dominated by the necessity to care for another family member who is sick or in pain. The effects of long-term illness or disability on a family can be devastating: in many cases, it happens to families who are already over-stressed, under-loved, and emotionally maxed out.

On the other hand, I have seen people who have been unemployed due to their pain or health condition choose to adopt new healthy habits: within a short period of time they are back at work making money, taking care of themselves and their families again, and are able to put away savings for their retirement.

I have heard every excuse you can imagine as to why people believe they can't afford the time or money to invest in their health. But the truth is that you must invest in your health today, or disease may bankrupt you in every way later. If you don't have the time and money to improve your health while you feel good, what makes you think you will have the time and money to improve your health once you have lost it? As Anthony Robbins once said, "you can make time for wellness now or you can make time for sickness later. The choice is yours."

With regard to your wellness, the three main ideas that I really want to drive home are: 1) health is not merely the absence of disease; 2) the body has an innate intelligence that runs a series of complex systems that rely on proper balance and coordination in order to function correctly; and 3) by living a wellness lifestyle, you can enrich your life with vibrant health. In the chapters that follow you will learn about the five components of wellness: alignment, exercise, nutrition, healthy thinking, and healthy lifestyle habits.

In addition, you will learn great strategies on how to create your own all-star wellness team, about our favorite essential wellness products, and how wellness is impacting America today and in the future.

SPECIAL SECTION

Perspectives on Wellness

By Dr. Jeffrey Spencer, M.A., D.C.

Wellness Chiropractor to the "world's greatest" athletes and performing artists, including Lance Armstrong, Tiger Woods, Troy Glaus, Bobby LaBonte, and U2.

Most people aren't living even close to their optimal potential. The insidious slow slide from youthful vitality and enthusiasm to diminished health is pandemic. A few pounds here, a little less activity there and 10-20 years down the line there's a completely transformed person barely resembling the former self in looks, performance, and optimism. It's a shock to confront that reality but the good news is, it is 100 percent reversible. What's inspiring to know is that, in most cases, a person's best work is always on the other side of life's worst moments.

For example, Lance Armstrong's spectacular Tour de France victories came after his near-death encounter with metastatic cancer. None of us are any different than Lance in that respect. Our lowest moments give us the opportunity to decide that we want to create a better life and provide empowerment to overcome great adversity.

Everyone at some point in their life will confront a period of long, sustained hardship, which in my experience has proven to be an essential rite of passage in developing the commitment, persistence, and passion necessary to express our birthright talents to the fullest and to appreciate life's gifts. Lance said it best when he said, "When you get a second chance, go all the way."

Each of us has our own "second chance": every second of our lives. Nobody in their right mind wants to live an ordinary, boring, and mediocre life when we have the ability to create an extraordinary life experience. In reality, it's next to impossible to make the commitment to "go all the way" in life or to manifest our highest talents before ill health or tragedy takes it from us, for it is the loss of health that creates the intimate knowledge that health is a gift.

Without our health, we are not capable of living a full life, let alone contributing constructively to others. Getting well is an individual process dependent on a person's state of health at the point of realization that life's present course doesn't have a future. It is by the realization that one's present state of life and health is no longer acceptable, that one finds the commitment to do what it takes to create a better life.

Discover Wellness Today; It Is Your Second Chance

As the wellness chiropractor to some of the world's greatest athletes, I have had the good fortune of seeing the amazing results of what a wellness lifestyle can do to enhance a person's health and performance. Thousands of chiropractors practice across America. They are all focused on providing great wellness care to people in their community; people who are seeking to improve their own health and well-being and live their very best life. Please know that you don't have to want to be the world's greatest athlete to benefit from living a wellness lifestyle.

Discover Wellness Recommends

The following list is a summary of the key items I've found that produce the best long-term results for my patients and myself:

1) It is of the utmost importance to ensure that the physical structure of your body is in proper alignment. Your spine and joints are the foundation of your body and are, by definition, the backbone of your body's

ability to function properly. I recommend that all of my top performing athletes, celebrities, and superstars receive consistent spinal care to ensure their optimal alignment and therefore their best health, performance, and well-being.

2) Do some form of cardiovascular training four to six days a week at low to moderate intensity for 30-60 minutes. Never overdo it, as this can lead to illness, injury, burnout, and increased inflammation in the body, which health experts agree is the gateway to all disease. If possible, the body prefers doing a few types of cardiovascular exercise throughout the week such as swimming, cycling, jogging, rowing, or walking.

3) Set the tone of the day by doing active strengthening and stretching exercises first thing in the morning, such as yoga, Tai Chi and Qi Gong, because they combine diaphragmatic breathing with movement. Doing this upon rising clears the mind and prepares the body for the day. People who do this have better attitudes than those who don't. Keep in mind that the body wasn't designed to exercise hard first thing in the morning.

4) The brain needs its own health and wellness program as much as the body does. It is well documented in scientific research that people who use their brains

regularly doing mental exercises are more productive than those who do not, and they are less prone to debilitating brain degenerative disease such as Alzheimer's. Chess, checkers, crossword puzzles, reading, and all forms of strategic planning and problem solving encourage brain fitness. Only a few minutes a day can do wonders.

5) The body is 70 percent water and this is where the chemical reactions that sustain life take place. Water plays a vital role in how cells talk to each other to orchestrate full body movement, overall health, and well-being. Most people are chronically dehydrated from not drinking enough pure water, not having enough minerals in the body, drinking too much coffee, and eating too many processed foods. As a general rule, eight glasses of pure water should be consumed per day. Water also helps detoxify disease-producing toxins from the environment such as air pollution, solvents, pesticides, paints, and home cleaners.

6) Take a multivitamin and mineral supplement daily to provide the micronutrients needed to support the body in today's rush-rush culture. Vitamins and minerals, however, are not a substitute for a diet rich in whole grains, vegetables, fruit, and non-farm raised fish and non-hormone or antibiotic-fed fowl or beef. Vitamins and minerals do not directly give us energy but

work with the food we eat for that purpose and should be viewed as a nutritional insurance policy.

7) Take an antioxidant supplement every day. Antioxidants are the vitamins A, C, E, and selenium, and are important for neutralizing the effects of molecules called free radicals that produce inflammation and accelerate aging in the body.

8) Every morning before going to work or interacting with people, invest a few deliberate minutes recommitting to your life's purpose. This anchors the spirit to the principles that will govern how you react to life and how you interact with other people.

9) Be charitable. People who help others seem to be happier and more optimistic than those who don't. There is something healthy about giving to others.

10) Mentors help shortcut life's learning curve and can make a powerful difference in a person's life. Giving back to humanity by mentoring empowers individuals and society. Be a mentor.

11) Always get enough rest. Refilling the energy stores from day to day is pivotal to being a long-term productive enthusiastic person. Excess fatigue creates

mental dullness and burnout. Being overly tired can make a person do and say things they deeply regret.

12) Never go too long without eating. Those who eat before getting hungry never deplete their energy stores that otherwise open the door for mental errors, injuries, and illness. Wellness depends on having a steady flow and regular supply of nutrients in the body to keep it and the mind strong and vital.

13) Resolve personal conflicts immediately. Being conflict-free allows the mind to explore more constructive life pursuits. It is well known that pent-up emotions are detrimental to health.

14) Building purposeful pause into daily life not only recharges the body, but the mind as well. More effort is not always better. Those who do not provide time for regular reflection are most often those who burn out the fastest and are least productive. A 15-20 minute break in the afternoon seems to be the magic formula to give the body that breather necessary to keep the brain and body moving at peak capacity.

15) Hobbies are a great way to keep passion in life, keep the mind alert and engaged, build another career, and free the mind from daily stresses and strains. All

of the most successful people I know do several things in life and never spend too much time at one thing too often, as that's what puts monotony in life. For example, I know a very successful doctor who also writes books, and an accountant whose passion is woodworking. Both of these people are some of the most vital people I've ever met.

16) Get enough sleep. It is the only way to recover from life's daily stresses and strains. Lack of sleep leads to poor recovery and eventually breaks the body down, resulting in needless injury or illness. A minimum of seven hours of sleep each night is recommended.

17) Staying well depends on breathing good air. Oxygen is the spark plug that generates our energy. To get the best quality air, spend time outdoors on a regular basis and use a high-quality air filter indoors.

18) Avoid exposure to air pollution, pesticides, moldy places, chemical sprays, and solvents, as they are poison to our bodies. The energy required to detoxify the body of toxins takes away from our productivity and increases our risk of illness by adding to the total body burden.

19) People living quality wellness lives cultivate and nourish meaningful relationships. Make it a priority to spend time with people who enrich your life and are of like mind. Having fun with your self, family, and friends, and being social are important in being well, and help make the world a better place.

Dr. Jeffery Spencer is, as described by Lance Armstrong in his book Every Second Counts, *"part doctor, part guru, part medicine.... While he fixed us physically he also fixed us mentally ... we believed Jeff could fix anything ... judging by the people in and out of his room the most important person on the team might have been Jeff." Dr. Spencer was Lance Armstrong's personal chiropractor at all seven of his Tour de France victories.*

To download Dr. Jeffrey Spencer's recommendations and to read more celebrity testimonials, visit DiscoverWellnessCenter.com

9

Alignment

People today are beginning to take more responsibility for their health and are asking better questions. They are far better informed and are demanding more from their doctors than ever before. People have raised the bar: they want more natural and more effective forms of health care for themselves and their loved ones. Today's health care consumers want to feel healthy and to feel good about themselves in the process. In addition, they are extremely loyal to health care professionals who demonstrate respect, concern, confidence, and compassion, and who deliver consistent, natural results. This trend reflects a growing dissatisfaction with conventional, sickness-based medical services and a dramatic move towards wellness care.

Alignment first and foremost refers to living in alignment with your core values and life purpose. Stress and the impact stress has on allowing for disease to manifest in your body often results from living with actions that are out of alignment with your values. Wellness expert Dr. Patrick Gentempo teaches that living in contradiction to your core values/life purpose always leads to destruction. It is vital to your health, well-being and quality of life to create a lifestyle that is in alignment with what's most important to you in life.

If your health is a priority for you and you do not live a lifestyle in alignment with that value, it will lead to health problems over time. If your marriage is of value to you and you do not live in alignment with the values of your marriage, it will lead to destruction of the marriage over time. If you value your family and you do not live in alignment with the responsibilities of your role in your family it will lead to destruction of your family. It is a natural law of life that your actions must be consistent or in alignment with your values to experience success in life.

Complementary health care acknowledges the body's innate intelligence. The term "mind-body connection" is frequently used in the popular press but is seldom defined. In fact, what connects the mind to the body is the nervous system, which medical textbooks refer to as the "master control system." You will be amazed at how the spine and nervous system are interrelated and connected to every aspect of our expression of health and wellness.

Breakdown between the brain and body will always be related to a nervous system malfunction. Any interference with the normal function of the nervous system will negatively affect

Secret to Your Wellness

Visit DiscoverWellnessCenter.com for our interactive 3-D animated demonstration of the mind-body connection.

The Nervous Sytem

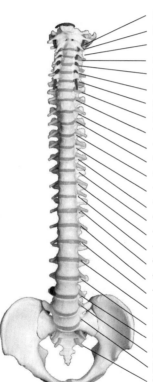

C1 • Virtually all organ systems in the body
C2 • Brain, eyes, sinuses
C3 • Eyes, Sinuses
C4 • Submaxillary and sublingual glands
C5 • Submaxillary, sublingual, and parotid glands
C6 • Parotid, sublingual, and thyroid glands
C7 • Thyroid gland and lungs
C8 • Thyroid, lungs, and heart
T1 • Thyroid, lungs, heart and carotid artery
T2 • Lungs, heart, and carotid artery
T3 • Lungs, heart, and stomach
T4 • Liver and stomach
T5 • Stomach
T6 • Pancreas
T7 • Spleen
T8 • Liver
T9 • Adrenals and kidneys
T10 • Small intestines and kidneys
T11 • Kidneys
T12 • Kidneys
L1 • Large intestine
L2 • Large intestine
L3 • Large intestine and bladder
L4 • Large intestine and bladder
L5 • Large intestine and bladder
Sacral • Large intestine and bladder

All of the functions related to the human body are controlled by the extensive neural network continually sending and receiving electrical impulses to and from the brain. Stress in any part of the nervous system may result in a variety of health problems throughout the body.

an individual's health and well-being. Conversely, anything that removes or reduces nervous system interference will help to improve an individual's health and quality of life.

The Four Pillars of a Healthy Spine

The human body is an amazingly complex system of bones, joints, muscles, and nerves, designed to work together to accomplish one thing: motion. Remember that motion is life. Everything about the human body is designed with motion in mind: nerve fibers stimulate the muscles to contract, muscles contract to move the bones, bones move around joints, and the nervous system controls it all.

As a matter of fact, research has shown that motion is so critical to our body's health that a lack of motion has a detrimental affect on everything from digestion to our emotional state, immune function, our ability to concentrate, how well we sleep, and even to how long we live. If your lifestyle does not include enough motion, your body cannot function efficiently. First, you will not be as physically healthy and will suffer from a wide variety of physical ailments, ranging from headaches to high blood pressure. Second, you will not be as productive in your life because of reduced energy levels and the lack of ability to mentally focus. Third, because you have less energy, your activity level will tend to drop off even further over time, creating a downward spiral of reduced energy and less activity until you get to a point where even the demands of a sedentary job leave you physically exhausted at the end of the day.

Pillar One: Posture

The ancient Japanese art form of growing Bonsai trees is fascinating. Bonsai trees are essentially normal shrubs that have been consistently stressed in a particular way for a long time to create a posture which would never be found in nature. Depending on how the tree is stressed while it grows, it may end up looking like a miniature version of a full-sized tree, or it may end up looking like a wild tangle of branches with twists and loops.

To most people, "good posture" simply means sitting and standing up straight. Few of us realize the importance of posture to our health and performance. The human body craves alignment. When we are properly aligned, our bones, not our muscles, support our weight, reducing effort and strain. The big payoff with proper posture is that we feel healthier, have more energy, and move gracefully. So while the word "posture" may conjure up images of book-balancing charm-school girls, it is not just about standing up straight. It's about being aware of and connected to every part of your self.

Posture ranks right up at the top of the list when you are talking about good health. It is as important as eating right, exercising, getting proper rest, and avoiding potentially harmful substances like alcohol, drugs, and tobacco. Maintaining a healthy posture minimizes the stress on your body due to gravity. Without good posture, you cannot really be physically fit, and can actually damage your spine every time you exercise.

Ideally, our bones stack up one upon the other: the head rests directly on top of the spine, which sits directly over the pelvis, which sits directly over the knees and ankles. But if you spend hours every day sitting in a chair, if you hunch forward or balance your weight primarily on one leg, the muscles of your neck and back have to carry the weight of the body, rather than it being supported by the spine. The resulting tension and joint pressure can affect you not only physically, but emotionally, too, —from the predictable shoulder and back pain to headaches, short attention span, and depression.

Poor posture distorts the alignment of bones, chronically tenses muscles, and contributes to stressful conditions such as loss of vital lung capacity, increased fatigue, reduced blood and oxygen to the brain, limited range of motion, stiffness of joints, pain syndromes, reduced mental alertness, and decreased productivity at work. According to the Nobel Laureate Dr. Roger Sperry, "The more mechanically distorted a person is, the less energy is available for thinking, metabolism, and healing."

The most immediate problem with poor posture is that it creates a lot of chronic muscle tension as the weight of the head and upper body must be supported by the muscles instead of the bones. This effect becomes more pronounced the further your posture deviates from your body's center of balance.

Secret to Your Wellness

Visit DiscoverWellnessCenter.com for our interactive 3-D animated demonstration of proper postures for driving, sitting, sleeping, and standing.

Healthy Posture

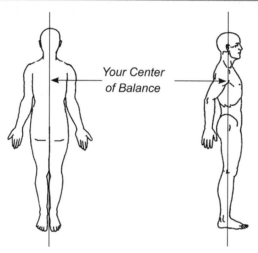

Your Center of Balance

Maintaining a healthy posture is critical for minimizing stress on your body. Whenever your posture deviates from your center of balance, your muscles have to bear the extra load and will become tight, painful, and inflamed.

To illustrate this idea further, think about carrying a briefcase. If you had to carry a briefcase with your arms outstretched in front of you, it would not take long before the muscles of your shoulders would be completely exhausted. This is because carrying the briefcase far away from your center of balance places undue stress on your shoulder muscles. If you held the same briefcase down at your side, your muscles would not fatigue as quickly, because the briefcase is closer to your center of balance and therefore the weight is supported by the bones of the skeleton, rather than the muscles.

In some parts of the world, women carry big pots full of water from distant water sources back to their homes. They are able to carry these heavy pots a long distance without significant effort because they balance them on the tops of their heads, thereby carrying the pots at their center of balance and allowing the strength of their skeletons to bear the weight, rather than their muscles.

Correcting bad posture and the physical problems that result can be accomplished in two ways. The first is by eliminating as much "bad" stress from your body as possible. Bad stress includes all the factors, habits, or stressors that cause your body to deviate from your structural center. Bad stress can result from a poorly adjusted workstation at work, from not having your seat adjusted correctly in your car, or even from carrying too much weight around in a heavy purse or backpack.

The second is by applying "good" stress on the body in an effort to move your posture back toward your center of balance. This is accomplished through a series of exercises, stretches, adjustments, and changes to your physical environment, all designed to help correct your posture. Getting your body back to its center of balance by improving your posture is critically important to improving how you feel.

Pillar Two: Movement

Imagine waking up one morning with a frozen shoulder where you couldn't move your upper arm more than a few inches in any direction. How much would that affect your ability to do your job? How much would that affect your ability to drive your car or even to dress yourself? How much would that affect your ability to concentrate on anything other than your shoulder? Obviously, if your shoulder did not move correctly, it would have a dramatic impact on your life. Well, the same is true with movement in every part of your body. If things aren't moving the way they are supposed to move, it will have a negative impact on your ability to function at work, take care of the demands of everyday life, and even your ability to concentrate.

Many people with severe low back pain report that their pain came on suddenly when they did something as simple as bend down to pet their cat, put on their socks, or pick up the newspaper. Just about everyone would agree that a person's body should be able to handle such simple movements. So what has happened?

In every one of these cases, the joints of the people's body were "all locked up"—they were barely moving at all. When the joints in one area of the body do not move the way they should, other areas of the body are forced to move more in order to compensate. This creates a significant stress on those areas that have to pick up the slack, and it soon leads to pain and inflammation. At the same time, the areas that don't have normal movement will slowly worsen as the muscles continue to tighten, the joints stick together, and the ligaments and tendons shorten. This leaves the body in a very unstable condition; if left unchecked, this process will continue until the body can hardly move at all. That is how a person comes to suffer flare-ups of pain at the slightest provocation.

Most of us have seen people who have lost most of their normal mobility—their bodies look like they have been starched stiff. This is especially prevalent among the elderly. Contrary to popular belief, however, this is not an inevitable effect of aging; rather it is the inevitable effect of not maintaining the body's mobility through exercise, healthy alignment, and body mechanics. There are people in their 60s, 70s, or even older, who are stronger and more flexible than the average person in their 30s, simply because they keep themselves exercising.

Maintaining mobility is critical in order to live free from pain and disability. Maintaining good mobility is not difficult, but it does not happen on its own. Just as with developing a good posture, it is necessary that you perform specific exercises and stretches to keep your muscles, ligaments, and tendons flexible and healthy. In addition, it is necessary that all of the joints in your body are kept moving correctly as well. This can be achieved to a great degree through the stretches and exercises in this book. Most people also find routine spinal adjustments to be very beneficial.

Pillar Three: Strength

Strong muscles keep your body upright and allow you to move. Good muscle strength and balance are critical to maintain proper posture and minimize muscle tension. Your muscles function much like the wires that hold up a tall radio or television antenna. If the wires are equally strong on all sides, the antenna will stand up straight. If one of the wires becomes weak or breaks, the antenna will either lean to the side or collapse. The same is true with your body. If the muscles on all sides of your spine are balanced and strong, your body will stand up straight and strong. Unfortunately, most people don't have balanced and strong muscles—due, once again, to lack of exercise and to misalignments of the spine.

Muscles are very efficient at getting stronger or weaker in response to the demands placed on them. Since most of us sit at a desk, drive a car, and sit on the sofa at home, many of our muscles are not challenged. Consequently, they become weak. At the same time, the muscles that are constantly used throughout the day become strong. This imbalance of muscle strength contributes to poor posture and chronic muscle tension. Left unchecked, muscle imbalances tend to get worse, not better, because of a phenomenon called "reciprocal inhibition."

Reciprocal inhibition literally means "shutting down the opposite." For all of the muscles that move your body in one direction, there are opposing muscles that move the body in the opposite direction. In order to keep these muscles from working against each other, when the body contracts one muscle group, it forces the opposing group to relax—it shuts down the opposite muscles. When consistently only one set of muscles is used, the opposing group, from being continuously shut down, is liable to atrophy.

This phenomenon is especially important to people who work at a desk, because all day long the same muscles in the upper back and chest area of the body are used. This means that all day long the body is essentially shutting down the opposite muscles in the middle back. Over time, the muscles in the middle back become very weak because they are not being worked like the muscles in the front of the body. This contributes to poor posture and chronic muscle spasms and pain.

Pillar Four: Balance

John was a powerlifter who was suffering from shoulder pain. He had x-rays and all of the normal tests in an attempt to figure out what was wrong with his shoulders, but everything turned up normal. He was young and healthy, had incredible strength, great flexibility, and no specific injury to the shoulders. However, since the shoulder is a very mobile and unstable joint, if all of its muscles are not in balance and contracting in the correct order or with the right amount of tension, the result can be increased mechanical stress of the shoulder joint, ultimately resulting in pain.

John's chiropractor recommended a series of very simple, lightweight exercises for John to do on a daily basis for the purpose of re-establishing normal shoulder coordination. John also received adjustments to improve the alignment and restrictions in his neck. The adjustments decreased the stress on the nerves affecting his shoulder muscles. The results were immediate and profound. Not only did John's pain completely disappear, but his ability to bench press improved. It turned out that John's only problem was that his muscles were not coordinating correctly. Although posture, joint mobility, and muscle strength are all important, they are not the whole story. We also must have a balanced, coordinated control over our muscles and joints if we want to enjoy good body mechanics.

Healthy balance is simply the result of using the body in the manner in which it was designed. Exercises such as walking, swimming, yoga, Pilates, bicycling, martial arts, and bodybuilding all help to improve muscle coordination, whereas working at a desk, reading, and watching television do the opposite. Without realizing it, most people are in a dramatic state of muscle incoordination. This occurs simply because they sit for many hours every day and do not perform regular exercises that will work to keep all of the muscles in their body properly coordinated. This muscular incoordination contributes to muscle tightness, restricted movement, and joint pain.

Spinal Misalignment: The Vertebral Subluxation Complex

The most vital structure of the body in maintaining proper alignment is the spine. The spine is the backbone or mainframe of the body. Your head sits on it, your arms and legs extend from it. It is also the main protector of your spinal cord, known as the tail of the brain. Therefore, if there is misalignment of the spine, it can and will negatively affect the structure and function of other parts of your body.

The word "subluxation" comes from the Latin words meaning "to dislocate" (luxare) and "somewhat" or "slightly" (sub). So the term "vertebral subluxation" literally means a slight dislocation (misalignment) of the bones in the spine. Another way of understanding the word "subluxation" is to recognize the word-roots "sub," meaning "below" (just as sub-marine means below the water), and "lux," meaning "light," which is the physiological expression of life. Life is light or electricity going through the nervous system animating our bodies, keeping us alive. Dr. Arno Burnier teaches that a subluxation can also be thought of as a condition of less light or of less life.

Either way you choose to think of the word subluxation, today's research has evolved our understanding of what a subluxation is. It includes a complex of neurological, structural, and functional changes that occur when a bone is misaligned. For this reason, chiropractors usually refer to a subluxation of the spine as a Vertebral Subluxation Complex, or VSC. The following are the five components that contribute to the Vertebral Subluxation Complex:

The Bone Component

This occurs where the vertebra is either out of position, not moving properly, or is undergoing degeneration. This frequently leads to a narrowing of the spaces between the bones through which the nerves pass, often resulting in compression of the discs and irritation or impingement of the nerve itself. People may notice a clicking or cracking sound or feel extra movement in their neck and back. Think of a bicycle chain that has two links rusting together. It will certainly affect the function of

 # Secret to Your Wellness

Visit DiscoverWellnessCenter.com for our interactive 3-D animated demonstration of the damaging effects of subluxations on the nervous system.

Subluxation

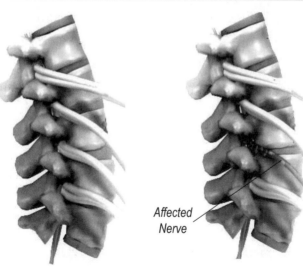

Affected Nerve

Normal   Subluxated

A vertebral subluxation refers to a spinal bone that has become misaligned. Pressure applied to nerves because of a subluxation can affect the proper function of all the organs in your body, and can lead to pain, weakness, and numbness.

the rest of the chain and will likely cause it to wear out much faster.

The Neurological Component

This is the disruption of the normal flow of energy along the nerve fibers, causing the messages traveling along the nerves to become distorted. The result is that all of the tissues fed by those nerves receive distorted signals from the brain and are not able to function normally. Over time, this can lead to a whole host of conditions, such as peptic ulcers, constipation, and other organ system dysfunction. You could think of this as the organs of your body receiving poor cell phone reception from the brain and then functioning improperly because they can't accurately understand what the brain is telling them to do. You can imagine the brain asking the organs of your body, "can you hear me now?"

The Muscular Component

Since nerves control the muscles that help hold the vertebrae in place, muscles have to be considered an integral part of the Vertebral Subluxation Complex. In fact, muscles both affect and are affected by the VSC. A subluxation irritates a nerve and the irritated nerve causes a muscle to spasm. The muscle in spasm then pulls the attached vertebrae further out of place, which further irritates the nerve and replays the cycle. In addition, as the muscles around a subluxation become inflamed and spasm, trigger points develop. Most people confuse subluxations with pulled or strained muscles, because the muscles are the body part in which people experience pain most. People don't feel their bones misaligned; they feel the pain in their muscles.

The Soft Tissue Component

The VSC will also affect the surrounding tendons, ligaments, blood supply, and other tissues as the misaligned vertebrae tug and squeeze the connective tissue with tremendous force. Over time, the soft tissues can become stretched or scarred, leaving the spine with either permanent instability or restriction. This is one of the components of the subluxation that take the longest to heal. That is why you may hear a chiropractor recommending restoration care, which goes beyond just the temporary relief of pain. Research has shown that it can take months, and in some cases years, for the soft tissue component of a subluxation to heal correctly.

The Degeneration Component

This describes the degeneration and decay that occurs to the spine due to the above four components. Some doctors mistakenly refer to this process as "normal" or "aging" because it is so common, but if you were to see degeneration on your spinal x-ray, you might ask yourself why the other vertebrae of your spine are not degenerating, since obviously they are all the same age.

Early spinal decay is often a result of poor spinal alignment that is left uncorrected. This is an important fact to keep in mind when considering whether to maintain your spinal alignment even when you are asymptomatic. Like heart disease and cancer, spinal degeneration is a silent process that does not announce itself until it has already developed.

An x-ray of your spine can be incredibly valuable here: you can differentiate a short-term misalignment from a long-term misalignment and care for it accordingly. Spinal degeneration is a progressive condition that continues to get worse over time if not properly cared for, leading to chronic pain, inflammation, arthritis, muscle trigger points, the formation of bone spurs and loss of movement, as well as muscle weakness and spasm.

Manual Manipulation

Manual manipulation of the spine and other joints in the body has been around for centuries. Ancient writings from China and Greece dating between 2700 BC and 1500 BC mention spinal manipulation and the maneuvering of the lower extremities to ease low back pain. Hippocrates, the famous Greek physician who lived from 460-357 BC, published a text detailing the importance of manual manipulation. In one of his writings he declares, "Get knowledge of the spine, for this is the requisite for many diseases." Evidence of manual manipulation of the body has been found among the ancient civilizations of Egypt, Babylon, Syria, Japan, the Incas, Mayans, and Native Americans. The understanding of the human frame or structure and its relationship to human function or health has been around since ancient times and is best described by the famous Thomas Edison quote: "The doctor of the future will give no medicine, but will interest his patients in the care of the human frame, in diet, and in the cause and prevention of disease."

Chiropractic: The Best Kept Secret in Health Care

The word "chiropractic" comes from the Greek words "cheir" (hand) and "praxis" (action), and literally means "done by hand." The official beginning of the chiropractic profession is dated to 1895 when Daniel David Palmer discovered the benefits of manually adjusting the spine. Two years later, in 1897, Dr. Palmer founded the Palmer School of Chiropractic in Davenport, Iowa, which continues to train doctors of chiropractic to this day.

Like conventional medicine, chiropractic is based upon scientific principles of (1) diagnosis through testing and observation and (2) providing care based upon the practitioner's rigorous training and clinical experience. Unlike conventional medicine, however, which focuses on attempting to treat disease once it occurs, chiropractic emphasizes improving the health of the individual in order to reduce the risk of pain and illness in the first place.

Most people would rather be healthy and avoid illness, if they could: this is one of the main reasons for the surge in the popularity of chiropractic care. People are recognizing the benefit of seeking a wellness chiropractor who will help them achieve and maintain optimal health proactively.

Chiropractors recognize that one of the main causes of pain and dis-ease is the misalignment and abnormal motion of the vertebrae in the spinal column, called a subluxation. Chiropractic works by adjusting the effects of these subluxations in the spine, thereby relieving pressure on and irritation of the nerves, restoring joint mobility, and returning the body back to a state of normal function.

More and more scientific research is demonstrating the tremendous detrimental effect that subluxations have on the health of the body. In order to be truly healthy, it is vital that your nervous system be functioning free of interference from subluxations. Just like a dentist is the specialist trained to care for your teeth or an optometrist is the specialist trained to care for your eyes, chiropractors are the specialists trained to care for your spine and nervous system, which influences all of the other systems of your body.

According to one study, *The Chiropractic Patient Satisfaction and Utilization*, people receiving long-term chiropractic care have taken less medication 71 percent of the time, have had an overall improvement in health 87 percent of the time, are living a healthier lifestyle 92 percent of the time, and have a decrease in pain 99 percent of the time.[1] These are powerful statistics that demonstrate why chiropractic care continues to be embraced by Americans.

Chiropractic patients enjoy increased flexibility, improved posture, improved or eliminated pain, a more relaxed and calm state, and an enhanced energy level—in short, an improved overall quality of life.

Numerous studies have demonstrated that chiropractic care is one of the most effective ways to help the body heal from back pain, neck pain, headaches, whiplash, sports injuries, and many other types of musculoskeletal problems. It has even been shown to be effective in reducing high blood pressure, decreasing the frequency of childhood ear infections (otitis media), and improving the symptoms of asthma.

Throughout the twentieth century, in spite of many years of prejudice, the profession of chiropractic has gained considerable recognition and scientific support. Research studies have clearly demonstrated the value of chiropractic care in reducing health care costs, improving recovery rates, and increasing patient satisfaction. In fact, a major study conducted in Canada, the "1993 Manga Study," concluded that chiropractic care would save hundreds of millions of dollars annually in work disability payments and direct health care costs.[2] Several major studies conducted by the US Government, the Rand Corporation, and others have all demonstrated the incredible value of chiropractic care.[3-5]

The chiropractic approach to health care is holistic, meaning that it addresses your overall health. The holistic approach considers the many lifestyle factors, such as exercise, diet, relaxation, rest, and your environment, that affect your health. For this reason, a wellness lifestyle—being mindful of your diet, exercise, relaxation, and sleeping habits—works hand in hand with chiropractic care. Unfortunately, there are still many people who have never been to a chiropractor and don't understand what we do.

What is Chiropractic Care?

Spinal adjustments to correct subluxations are what make doctors of chiropractic unique in comparison with any other type of health care professional. The term "adjustment" refers to the specific force chiropractors apply to vertebrae that have abnormal movement patterns or fail to function normally. The objective of the chiropractic adjustment is to reduce the subluxation, which results in an increased range of motion, reduced nerve irritability, reduced muscle spasm, reduced pain, and improved function.

The chiropractic adjustment is a quick thrust applied to a vertebra for the purpose of correcting its position, movement, or both. Adjustments are often accompanied by an audible release of gas in the spinal joints that sounds like a "crack." The sound sometimes surprises people the first time they get adjusted, but the sensation is usually relieving. Occasionally, minor discomfort is experienced, especially if the surrounding muscles are in spasm or the person tenses up during the chiropractic procedure. This is often due to either significant muscle tightness or the person having a hard time relaxing during their adjustments. There are times when the audible "cracking" does not occur. Some adjusting techniques are designed to move the spine in a way that does not produce the audible sound at all.

Chiropractic is so much more than simply a means of relieving pain. Ultimately, the goal of receiving adjustments should be to restore the body to its natural state of optimal health. In order to accomplish this, chiropractors can use and recommend a variety of natural healing methods, including adjustments, massage, trigger point therapy, nutrition, exercise rehabilitation, and counseling on lifestyle issues that impact your health. The primary focus is simply to remove those things which interfere with the body's natural normal healing ability.

The adjustment of the spine is the primary objective of a chiropractor. There are some chiropractors who also adjust the extremities and use other forms of physiological therapeutics including the use of electrical stimulation, ultrasound, traction, neuromuscular re-education, and a variety of manual therapies. Increasingly, chiropractors' offices are becoming full-service wellness centers providing a variety of wellness services.

A new trend that chiropractic wellness centers offer is wellness coaching. Some programs offer coaching at the wellness center, while others offer wellness coaching via telephone, email, or online instant messenger in an effort to make it more convenient. Chiropractic wellness centers may offer seminars in a variety of subjects such as spinal alignment, improved posture, and ergonomics, as well as programs on weight management, relaxation, smoking cessation, nutrition, and exercise. Some even offer prenatal and postnatal healthy baby programs. The increasing number of chiropractic centers providing extensive wellness programs makes it convenient and affordable for just about anyone to adopt a wellness lifestyle.

Chiropractors are doctors who understand that within each of us is an innate wisdom or healthy energy that will express itself as perfect health and well-being if we allow it to. Therefore, the focus of chiropractic care is to remove any physiological blocks to the proper expression of the body's innate wisdom. Once these interferences are reduced, improved health is the natural consequence. Who wouldn't want that?

Three Phases of Chiropractic Care

Providing chiropractic care is like building a house: certain things have to happen in a particular order in order for everything to stand strong and work correctly. When building a house, if you tried to put up your walls before you had a solid foundation, your walls would be weak and eventually collapse. If you tried to put on your roof before the walls were ready, you would run into the same problem. The same is true for your body. Your body has to go through a particular plan of care in order to repair itself correctly and fully. There are three general phases of chiropractic care: 1) relief care, 2) corrective/restorative care, and 3) wellness care.

Phase One - Relief Care

Some people first go to a chiropractor because they are in pain. In this first phase of care, the main goal is to reduce the symptoms. Sometimes this will require daily visits, or two to three visits per week for an initial series of visits.

The Three Phases of Chiropractic Care

Phase 1	Phase 2	Phase 3
Relief Care	**Corrective Care**	**Wellness Care**
The first objective is to help you feel better. During this phase, the goal is to relieve pain.	During the corrective care phase, muscles and other tissues are allowed to heal more completely, thereby helping to prevent re-injury.	Once your body has fully healed, it is important to come in for periodic adjustments to improve your well-being.

Most people are under the assumption that if they don't feel any pain, then there is nothing wrong with them. Unfortunately, pain is a very poor indicator of health. In fact, pain and other symptoms frequently only appear after a disease or condition has become advanced. Consider a cavity in your tooth. Does it hurt when it first develops or only after it has become serious? How about cancer? Whether you are talking about cancer, heart disease, diabetes, stress, or problems with the spine, pain is usually the last thing to appear. When you begin chiropractic care, pain is also the first symptom to disappear, even though much of the underlying condition remains.

Phase Two - Corrective/Restorative Care

Most chiropractors regard the elimination of symptoms as the easiest part of a person's care. If all the chiropractor does is reduce the pain and stop there, the chances of the condition recurring are much greater. In order to prevent a rapid recurrence of symptoms, it is necessary to continue care even after the symptoms are gone.

During the corrective/restorative phase of care, you will not have to receive adjustments as often as during the first phase of care, and, depending on your particular circumstances, you may begin doing exercises and stretches either at the center or at home to help accelerate your healing. Do not be discouraged if you have mild flare-ups in your symptoms on occasion. This is normal. Flare-ups are bound to occur during this phase because the body has not fully healed. Depending on the severity of your injury or condition and how long you have been suffering from it, this phase of your care may last anywhere from a few months to a couple of years.

Phase Three - Wellness Care

Once your body has healed, routine chiropractic checkups can help ensure that your physical problems do not return, and can help keep your body in optimal condition. Just like continuing an exercise program in order to sustain the benefits, it is necessary to continue chiropractic care to maintain and continually improve the health of your musculoskeletal system. When you make routine chiropractic care a part of your lifestyle, you avoid many of the aches and pains that so many people suffer, your joints last longer, and you are able to engage in more of the activities you love.

Spinal misalignments are much like diabetes, in that you can't just treat them once and expect everything to be better.

You must take care of yourself on a regular basis to remain healthy. Just as with diabetes, if you neglect to take care of your spine, over time your health will suffer—usually without any symptoms, until the problems have become severe. This is why I often call spinal subluxation "diabetes of the spine." It's not to say that your spine has diabetes but rather to drive home the idea that in order to keep your body well, it is critical to maintain your spine's alignment on a consistent basis.

Myths and Facts about Chiropractic

As successful as chiropractic has become, there are a lot of myths circulating among the general public. Times have definitely changed for the better, but the fact is that many people still do not understand what chiropractors do. Let's talk about a few of the more common myths about chiropractic.

Myth #1 - Chiropractors are not real doctors.

A chiropractic college grants a D.C. or Doctorate of Chiropractic degree. Chiropractors are licensed as health care providers in every US state and dozens of countries around the world. While the competition for acceptance to chiropractic school is not as fierce as medical school, the chiropractic and medical school curricula are extremely rigorous and virtually identical. In fact, chiropractors have more hours of classroom education than their medical counterparts. As part of their education, chiropractic students also complete a residency working with real clients in a clinical setting, supervised by licensed doctors of chiropractic. Once chiropractic students graduate, they have to pass four sets of national board exams, as well as state board exams in the states where they want to practice.

Chiropractors are professionals who are subject to the same type of testing procedures, licensing, and monitoring by state and national peer-reviewed boards as medical doctors are. Federal and state programs, such as Medicare, Medicaid, and Workers' Compensations programs, cover chiropractic care, and all federal agencies accept sick-leave certificates signed by doctors of chiropractic. Chiropractors are also commissioned as officers in the military.

The biggest difference between chiropractors and medical doctors lies not in their level of education, but in their preferred method of caring for people. Medical doctors are trained in the use of medicines (chemicals that affect your internal biochemistry) and surgery. Consequently, if you have a chemical problem, such as diabetes, hypothyroidism, or an infection, medical doctors can be very helpful. However, if your problem is that your spine is misaligned or you have soft tissue damage causing pain, there is no chemical in existence that can fix it.

You need a physical solution to correct a physical problem. That is where chiropractic really shines. Chiropractors provide physical solutions—adjustments, exercises, stretches, muscle therapy—to help the body heal from conditions that are physical in origin, such as back pain, muscle spasms, headaches, and poor posture. Another distinction is the fact that it is completely appropriate to receive chiropractic care even if you do not have symptoms. Unlike standard medical doctors, whom you visit when you have a symptom to be treated, chiropractors offer adjustments to improve spinal alignment and overall well-being before symptoms develop.

Myth #2 - Medical doctors don't like chiropractors.

The American Medical Association's opposition to chiropractic was at its strongest in the 1940s under the leadership

Chiropractic and Medical Education

Subject	Chiropractic Schools Total Hours	Medical Schools Total Hours
Anatomy	456	215
Biochemistry	161	100
Microbiology	145	145
Neurology	149	171
Physiology	243	174
Pathology	296	507
Psychology	56	323
Radiology	271	13
Orthopedics	168	2
Diagnosis	408	113
Obstetrics / Gynecology	66	284
Total Hours	**2,419**	**2,047**

(Based on the average curriculum of 18 chiropractic colleges and 22 medical schools)

of Morris Fishbein. Fishbein called chiropractors "rabid dogs" and referred to them as "playful and cute, but killers." He tried to portray chiropractors as members of an unscientific cult who cared about nothing but taking their patients' money. Up to the late 1970s and early 1980s, the medical establishment purposely conspired to try to destroy the profession of chiropractic. In fact, a landmark lawsuit in the Supreme Court of Illinois in the 1980s found that the American Medical Association was guilty of conspiracy and was ordered to pay restitution to the chiropractic profession.

In the years since, the opinion of most medical doctors has changed: several major studies have shown the superiority of chiropractic in helping people with a host of conditions, and medical doctors developed a better understanding as to what chiropractors actually do. Many people have returned to their medical doctors and told them about the great results they experienced at their chiropractor's office. Hospitals across the country now have chiropractors on staff, and many chiropractic offices have medical doctors on staff. Chiropractors and medical doctors are now much more comfortable working together in cases where medical care is necessary as an adjunct to chiropractic care.

Myth #3 - Once you start going to a chiropractor, you have to keep going for the rest of your life.

This statement comes up frequently when the topic of chiropractic is discussed. It is only partially true. You only have to continue going to the chiropractor as long as you wish to maintain the health of your neuromusculoskeletal system. Going to a chiropractor is much like going to the dentist, exercising at a gym, or eating a healthy diet: as long as you keep it up, you continue to enjoy the benefits.

Many years ago, dentists convinced everyone that the best time to go to the dentist is before your teeth hurt, and that routine dental care will help your teeth remain healthy for a long time. The same is true of chiropractic care for your spine. It is important to remember that, just like your teeth, your spine experiences normal wear and tear as you walk, drive, sit, lift, sleep, and bend. Routine chiropractic care can help you feel better, move with more freedom, and stay healthier throughout your lifetime. Although you can enjoy the benefits of chiropractic care even if you receive care for a short time, the real benefits come into play when you make chiropractic care a part of your wellness lifestyle.

Myth #4 - I don't need to see a chiropractor because I can crack my own neck and back.

Many chiropractors hear people claim that they can adjust themselves and watch as someone tries to demonstrate by putting their hands on their head and chin, and then thrusting to get an audible cracking sound. "See I can crack my own neck," they often say, thinking they are saving money every time they do it. Although it is true you can make your spine make noise, it is a myth that you can accurately correct your own subluxations by twisting your own neck or back when you feel uncomfortable. Although you may experience temporary relief, until the correct vertebrae are adjusted, you will only make the problem worse.

Frequently Asked Questions

Q: How can I tell if I need to see a chiropractor?

There are several ways you can test yourself and family members to determine whether you should go to a chiropractor for an evaluation:

- *Check your posture in the mirror. If you see that your head tilts, one of your shoulders is higher than the other or one of your hips is higher than the other, this often indicates that you are misaligned.*

- *Lie face down and ask someone to look at your heels to see if they are even. If one leg is contracted or shorter than the other, this often means that you are misaligned.*

- *Feel your neck and shoulders: do the muscles feel relaxed and at ease? Compare the muscle tone of your neck and shoulders to the muscle tone of your bicep when it is relaxed. If your neck and shoulders feel tense, you likely have unnecessary spinal stress.*

- *Turn your head to the right and then to the left. Do they turn equally far? Does one side appear to be more restricted than the other? Ask someone to watch you do it, and ask if they notice whether you can turn more to one side than the other.*

Other indications that you may need to see a chiropractor include:

- *Hearing sounds in your neck or back when you move*
- *Uneven wear in the heels of your shoes*
- *One of your feet flaring out when you walk*
- *Aches or pains in your head, neck, shoulders, arms, mid-back, low back, or down your legs*

If you are unsure, I recommend going to a chiropractor for an initial evaluation and letting them give you their professional opinion about your alignment. Ultimately, wouldn't it be great for them to analyze your alignment and tell you what good posture you have, and in what good health you are? If they do find misalignments, when do you think would be the best time to start realigning your spine?

Q: What should I expect at my chiropractic appointment?

Consultation

On your first visit to the office you will be welcomed and often given a brief tour of the office. Many people have never been to a chiropractor's office, and once they see how professional the atmosphere is, they feel much more relaxed. Your first visit is designed for the doctor to learn more about you, your condition, and your expectations to determine whether chiropractic care will help you meet your goals. Wellness chiropractors will ask you questions about your lifestyle habits and personal goals.

Examination

After your consultation, you will have an examination. This may include testing your reflexes and your ability to turn and bend, as well as other standard orthopedic, neurologic, postural, and physical examinations. The doctor may use advanced technologies to better understand the condition of your spine and nervous system, such as a Subluxation Station EMG, thermography, inclinometry, muscle testing, and more. If necessary, the doctor may take x-rays or refer you for additional testing procedures, such as an MRI or NCV test.

X-rays

X-rays are sometimes required to get a full evaluation of a client. The need for x-rays is considered on a case-by-case basis. X-rays are very valuable to actually visualize your spine. Most people are amazed once they see their x-rays and can often immediately identify their own misalignments and degeneration.

Report of Findings

Once all the information and examinations have been performed, the doctor will give you a report of findings and answer the three most popular questions: 1) Can you help me? 2) What do you recommend that I do to get better? 3) How much is this going to cost? Often the report of findings is done on the second visit, in order to allow time for the x-rays to be developed and analyzed, as well as to verify your insurance and put together a recommended action plan for you.

Recommended Action Plan

After discussing your health history and your personal goals, examining your spine, and reviewing any x-rays or tests, the doctor will discuss his or her recommendations with you. If you have a condition that requires care with other specialists, the doctor will make the appropriate referrals. If the doctor believes that chiropractic can help you, she/he will recommend a course of care. Many will also recommend the products that will best help you reach your goals.

Receiving Care

Most people begin to experience benefits from the very first adjustment. The adjustment is interactive, so you can express any concerns you have and discover the style of adjustment with which you will be most comfortable.

Q: What is a chiropractic adjustment?

The chiropractic adjustment is a gentle, quick thrust to a particular joint, typically in the spine, intended to restore normal position and movement. Adjustments are important for releasing adhesions in the joint and reducing stress on the nervous system. Because the nervous system is the master controller of all muscles and organs in the body, reducing stress on the nervous system through chiropractic adjustments will frequently lead to improved health in the entire body.

Q: How many adjustments will I need?

The total number of adjustments you need depends on five main factors: 1) your age, 2) your overall health, 3) the severity of your condition, 4) how long you have had your condition, and 5) what your ultimate goals are. If you are young, in good health, and have a mild condition that occurred very recently, you will need far fewer adjustments than if you are older, in poor general health, and have been struggling with a problem for many years. The total number of adjustments you will need also depends on whether you are interested in merely reducing immediate pain or in creating optimal long-term health.

Q: Will adjustments hurt?

Usually not. Some patients experience mild soreness after being adjusted, but this is the exception. Most people feel better very quickly after being adjusted.

Q: Will there be any side effects?

People may or may not experience side effects from chiropractic care. Effects may include temporary discomfort in parts of the body that were adjusted, headache, or tiredness. These effects tend to be minor and to resolve within one to two days. More commonly people express positive side effects, meaning they come in with the intention to heal from one particular condition, such as neck pain, and soon find out that their low back pain and menstrual cramps have decreased in frequency and intensity as well.

Q: How old should you be to see a chiropractor?

Improved spinal alignment can be beneficial to people of all ages. It only makes sense that if you have a spine, you should see a spinal expert who is trained to help you keep your spine healthy. Many people bring their newborn babies to get their spines checked for misalignments due to the stress and trauma of the birth process. Often very gentle adjustments can correct subluxations from birth and help a baby's healthy growth. It doesn't make any sense to wait until you are older and suffering with pain to start care when a problem could have been corrected when it was small.

Q: Do all chiropractors provide the same type of care?

Chiropractors often specialize based on their personal preferences and training, just like lawyers and medical doctors. Some like to focus their practice on pain relief, while others like to provide wellness care. Some like to provide care to families; some like to specialize in sports injuries, pediatrics, or geriatrics; and some specialize in specific techniques. It is often a good idea to ask questions and do some research to determine whether a specific doctor will be able to provide you with the care that best suits your needs.

Q: Do I still need to see the chiropractor
if my pain is gone?

It is very common for pain to disappear long before the correction of your condition is attained. As discussed earlier in this chapter, pain is not a very good indicator of health. Often, people are completely unaware of problems that are developing in their bodies. The point is that just because you are no longer experiencing pain does not mean that your problem no longer exists. It is important to continue receiving adjustments so that the underlying cause of the pain can be corrected.

Routine chiropractic care is one of the simplest ways to maintain and even improve the health of your body. Numerous research studies have shown that people who receive routine chiropractic care suffer fewer illnesses, injuries, and degenerative diseases, and report a better overall quality of life. In spite of the health benefits of chiropractic care, many people have never been to a chiropractor, most often because of fear coupled with a misunderstanding as to what chiropractic care is all about.

Q: Is chiropractic care safe during pregnancy?

Yes. It is very safe for both mother and baby. Most chiropractors spend many hours training to adjust the spines of pregnant women and many chiropractic adjusting tables have special modifications for pregnant women.

Q: Is chiropractic care safe for babies?

Yes. I am frequently asked by my pregnant patients to give the infant a spinal checkup soon after birth. This is because the birthing process can be traumatic for the infant and can cause very serious subluxations in the spine.

Q: Can chiropractors prescribe medication?

Chiropractors do not prescribe medications, although they may refer a patient to another provider for prescription medication if it is deemed necessary. In most cases, however, patients are better off with physical, rather than chemical, solutions for physical problems.

Makes sense doesn't it?

It has been said that the definition of insanity is to do the same thing repetitively and expect a different result. America has been focused on treating disease with medicines and surgery and has not invested much time in inspiring people to be proactive about their well-being. In fact, historically, doctors have been skeptical about the health benefits of natural healing methods because they do not fit the traditional diagnosis and treatment model of disease.

Hopefully, this chapter has provided enough information to illustrate a methodology that is new for many but makes a lot of sense to most. This may be the first time many of you are reading about how spinal alignment plays such a vital role in your health and well-being. Will this new information help you start a new path of wellness with a professional who has long awaited the opportunity to serve you?

SPECIAL SECTION

Perspectives on Wellness

By Dr. Gerry Clum, D.C.
President
Life Chiropractic College West

Wellness is one of those interesting topics that sound a little bit new-age and a little bit like grandma's common sense! Whether you view the concept of wellness as a revolutionary thought or the revival of age-old wisdom, one thing is for sure—wellness is about the journey, not the destination. There is another absolute about wellness that is important to put on the table right from the start: wellness is about the state of the person. It is far more than simply being healthy—as if that was a simple process! It is about physical, mental, social, and spiritual well-being. Wellness is not arrogant, conde-scending, or pompous in the direction of those who do not enjoy robust health and vitality. Wellness is about every day of our lives—the good ones, the poor ones, the greatest ones, and the worst ones. Wellness is about how we live our lives and how we make sense and give meaning to all of the vicissitudes of life.

Many of the strategies offered in these next chapters will be directed toward helping you gain physical capacity, strength, and resilience. Let's be clear, these are very good qualities to have, and to have them in great abundance is even better. But the goal is to help you gain insight and meaning into the circumstances of your life, and then to help you put your life to work for the betterment of the human condition. That may be the mother who better prepares her children for the world they will live in as adults. It may be the businessman who sees the greater good and the greater harm that stem from his immediate decisions, and then chooses to do what is best for the long term of all involved. It may be the politician or community leader who understands the awesome potential his or her respective group, organization, community, or culture possesses and acts in the best interest of the greater good for humankind.

It has been said, "To whom much is given, much is expected." Wellness is not a free ride. It requires hard work, attention to detail, and persistence beyond imagining. What we contribute to our society through the good fortune of our wellness is one example — an example of how life can be lived to achieve more than our wildest imaginations could have ever dreamt. Whether you are a health care provider, a health advocate, a person desiring to live a better, fuller life, or just a curious soul, the concepts of wellness dutifully applied will cause you to do a better job, be a better person, and offer a greater example.

One of the earliest authors and proponents of the concept of wellness in the 20th century was Don Ardell, Ph.D. Dr. Ardell continues to write passionately about the concept and pursuit of wellness. One of the most important contributions he has offered to this discussion involves the characteristics of the "wellest of the well." He offers the following as signs for how we should recognize these paragons of wellness:

- *High self-esteem and a positive outlook*
- *A foundation philosophy and a sense of purpose*
- *A strong sense of personal responsibility*
- *A good sense of humor and plenty of fun in life*
- *A concern for others and a respect for the environment*
- *A conscious commitment to personal excellence*
- *A sense of balance and an integrated lifestyle*

*• Freedom from addictive behaviors of a negative
or health-inhibiting nature*
*• A capacity to cope with whatever life presents
and to continue to learn*
• Grounded in reality
• Highly conditioned and physically fit
• A capacity to love and an ability to nurture
*• A capacity to manage life's demands and
communicate effectively*

A quick review of these characteristics reveals some very important insights: health care providers have little to do with achieving these circumstances and for the most part they are matters of mental perspective as opposed to physical capacity. Quite simply, we can attain great physical prowess and not be very "well" at all. Conversely, we can be quite ill, on our deathbeds even, and demonstrate almost all of the characteristics of the "wellest of the well."

Viewed from another perspective, we can consider the thoughts of Richard Smith, editor of one of the world's largest, oldest and most respected journals in health care, the *British Medical Journal* (BMJ). In a 2002 editorial about the arts, health care, health costs, and health care delivery systems, Smith posed a very provocative question: "Is it possible to be severely disabled, in pain, close to death, and in some sense 'healthy'?" His conclusion was simple and unequivocal: "I believe it is." Smith went on to note, "Health has to do with adaptation and acceptance. We will all be sick, suffer loss and hurt, and die. Health is not to do with avoiding these givens but with accepting them, even making sense of them."

Smith's discussion calls to mind Stephen Hawking, Ph.D., the world's foremost theoretical physicist, who has lived for decades in a wheelchair and communicated through a computerized speech synthesizer as a result of the ravages of Amyotrophic Lateral Sclerosis (ALS), also known as Lou Gehrig's Disease. Hawking continues to lecture, research, learn, teach, and grow. On his Web site he relates, "I am quite often asked 'How do you feel about having ALS?' The answer is, 'Not a lot.' I try to lead as normal a life as possible and not think about my condition or regret the things it prevents me from doing, which are not that many." Please remember he lives in a wheelchair, has nursing services 24 hours a day, communicates through a computer, and he will eventually die a premature death from ALS!

Stephen Hawking is healthier and displays more of the characteristics of wellness than most of the people you and I will encounter in our lives this week! Has

Hawking been called upon or offered the opportunity to "adapt" more than most in this life? I would say, yes. Has he also had to accept more about this life than most? Again I would say, yes.

Please allow me to offer one more illustration. This comes from the book *Chasing Darkness* written by Eugene O'Kelley. Mr. O'Kelley died in 2005 from a brain tumor known as an Astrocytoma Multiforme. He had approximately 100 days to "unwind" his life as a middle-aged chief executive officer with one of the world's most respected accounting firms, KPMG, a Fortune 500 corporation. In *Chasing Darkness*, O'Kelley offers how he dealt with the reality of his life and describes the process of acceptance and adaptation to this sudden development. Like an accountant, he went about the end of life with great precision and orderliness. He related working from the outer circle of his world, those with whom he had the least bond and tie, to the inner circle, those who formed the core of his life—his family and closest friends. He chronicled his movement through these concentric circles of attachment down to last moments of his life. His effort was capped by his wife, at his request, following his death.

In the tragedy of his early death he managed to leave a perspective about being "healthy" and demonstrating "wellness" down to his last breath. Was there sorrow, sadness, grief, despair? I am confident it was present in Herculean measure. But those factors did not rule the day. His "well-being" continued throughout—past and beyond his illness.

As you consider the strategies you will undertake to enhance the level of wellness in your life, please understand that your efforts, while in a very real sense a matter of enlightened self-interest, are in fact in service to humankind. The more fully and the "weller" you live your life, so, too are the lives around you—near and far—fuller, more rewarding, and richer. Thank you for your pursuit of wellness. It is a pleasure to be a fellow traveler with you along this lifelong path.

10

Exercise

Everyone knows that exercise is important for good health. Study after study has shown that exercise is effective at decreasing pain, reducing stress, improving immune function, lowering blood pressure, improving cardiac function, boosting energy, improving sleep, and maintaining a healthy body weight. The fact remains that although most people are aware of how important exercise is to their health, they still do not exercise in a way that maximizes the benefits available from exercise.

In their landmark book entitled *Biomarkers*, medical researchers Dr. William Evans and Dr. Irwin Rosenberg identified nine characteristic changes that occur as we age: a loss of muscle mass, a decrease in strength, a decrease in basal metabolic rate, a decrease in aerobic capacity, an increase in blood pressure, a loss of normal insulin action, a decrease in circulating HDL to total cholesterol ratio, a loss of bone density, and a decreased ability to control your body temperature. Each one of these measures of physical health tends to decline as we age. What Evans and Rosenberg discovered is that exercise was effective in reversing every single one of these symptoms of aging!

To those of the Baby Boomer generation, the name Jack La Lanne is synonymous with fitness. He hosted his own exercise television show for 34 years beginning in the early 1960s. Jack La Lanne was a sugar-addicted weakling for most of his youth, and at one point the family doctor told his parents that Jack may not have very long to live due to his ill health. That all changed on the day Jack decided he was going to quit eating junk food and begin exercising.

Over the ensuing years Jack accomplished what many would consider impossible feats, such as performing 1,033 push-ups in 23 minutes on national television at the age of 42, and on his 70th birthday, swimming 1.5 miles in San Francisco Bay while pulling 70 boats! At 93 years of age, he still exercises for two hours every day: one hour of swimming and one hour of weightlifting.

You don't have to exercise as intensely as Jack La Lanne in order to enjoy the benefits of exercise. But you do have to get up and get your body moving at least five or six days per week. The recommended exercise routine features a combination of aerobic exercise for the cardiovascular system and strength training for the musculoskeletal system. This will not only help you feel better and have more energy, it will also help to stabilize and strengthen your whole body.

Aerobic Exercise

Aerobic means "using oxygen." Aerobic exercises are those which utilize oxygen during the activity. Aerobic exercise trains the body to utilize oxygen more efficiently and improves overall cardiovascular fitness. Aerobic activities are those that are performed for an extended period of time at a low to medium intensity. Examples of aerobic activities are biking, aerobic walking, swimming, jogging, in-line skating, aerobic dance, cross-country skiing, and using an elliptical trainer. The benefits of aerobic activity include:

- *Improved breathing*
- *Increased energy throughout the day*
- *Improved heart health and cardiac output*
- *Decreased blood pressure*
- *Decreased serum cholesterol*
- *Decreased stress*
- *More restful sleep*
- *Improved mood and mental functioning*
- *Improved digestion and bowel function*

For maximum benefit, you should engage in at least 20 minutes of aerobic activity five or six days per week. If you can already do more than this, great! For those who have not engaged in regular activity for a while, even 20 minutes a day will be an accomplishment.

During aerobic exercise, you should be able to carry on a conversation without feeling too winded. If you are breathing too heavily to carry on a conversation easily, you should ease up a bit. As you become healthier, you will be able to increase the intensity of your activity without feeling short of breath.

This brings up another important point: a concept called the overload principle. The overload principle simply states that in order for you to benefit from physical activity, the intensity has to be greater than your body is used to. Only by pushing your body a little bit—by "overloading" it—will you enable your body to grow stronger. For example, if you have been taking the same walk around your block for a while, you might notice that it is no longer challenging; your body has adapted to this stimulus. To overload your cardiovascular system, you can try increasing either the intensity or duration of your exercise, or both. By walking faster and completing your walk at a more brisk pace, you make it more intense, and this will change the stimulus. Or you can do your walk twice, which means you would be exercising your cardiovascular system for a longer duration.

Strength Training

Strength training differs from aerobic training in three important ways. First, strength training involves activities that are more intense and much shorter in duration than aerobic activity—for example doing push-ups or sit-ups. Second, while aerobic training primarily improves the health of your cardio-vascular system, strength training improves the health of your muscles, bones, and joints. Third, while aerobic activity should be performed almost every day for maximum benefit, you only need to engage in strength training two to three times per week in order to maximize the effects of training. The benefits of strength training include:

- *Increased muscle and bone strength*
- *Improved muscle tone and body shape*
- *Improved hormone function*
- *Improved mood and mental functioning*
- *Increased weight loss*
- *Decreased serum cholesterol*
- *Decreased stress*
- *More restful sleep*
- *Increased metabolism*

To benefit from strength training, it is not necessary that you spend long grueling hours in the gym every day. In fact, you can experience a significant improvement in your strength and muscle tone by weightlifting for one hour just two or three times a week!

The key to successful strength training is the same as aerobic exercise—intensity and duration—but applied in a slightly different way. The harder you work your muscles during your strength workouts, the quicker you will see improvements.

Each time you exercise your muscles hard and overload them, your body goes to work to build more muscle. As long as you continue to slowly increase the weight that you use week after week and consistently reinforce this stimulus two to three times a week, your muscles will continue to grow in strength. Most people begin to see a difference in their strength and how they look after a few weeks of strength training.

Stretching

Stretching not only feels great, it is also very effective at reducing muscle tension, decreasing stress, and maintaining flexibility and joint mobility. In order to experience the benefits of stretching, however, it is important that you stretch correctly. Stretching your muscles too hard, bouncing while holding a stretch, or stretching your muscles when they are too cold can injure your muscles and lead to muscle tightness. Proper stretching technique is easy, provided you follow a few simple rules.

The first rule is to never stretch your muscles too hard. You should only stretch to the point where you feel a mild pull on the muscle. If you attempt to stretch further, you may cause small muscle tears and create a reflex tightening of the muscle. Repetitive overstretching can cause scarring of the muscle and a loss of flexibility.

The second rule is to never bounce while stretching. When you bounce, you momentarily force your muscles to overstretch;

this causes the muscle to automatically reflex in an attempt to protect itself and can increase your risk of muscular injury.

The third rule is to only stretch your muscles when they are warm. Muscles are a lot like plastic. If you heat plastic, you can bend it and stretch it without breaking it. By stretching only after you are warmed up, you will make your stretching much more safe and effective.

Individual Exercises and Stretches

In the pages that follow you will find exercises and stretches recommended to help people recover from injury and maintain their optimal health. Before trying these exercises by yourself, be sure to check with your chiropractor to ensure that you can do them safely.

The Dumbbell Row

The Dumbbell Row is without question the best overall upper back exercise you can do. It not only develops your rhomboid muscles very well, but it is also a powerful exercise to recoordinate all of the muscles of the upper and mid-back. It also improves the motion in the entire back and encourages proper posture.

Although this is not a difficult exercise to do, many people find it difficult at first because their upper back muscles are not coordinated. If the Dumbbell Row is done correctly, you should feel the muscles between your shoulder blades getting a good workout. But don't be alarmed if you don't feel anything at first or if you feel it more in your arms. As the muscles in your upper back begin to fire correctly, you should feel the muscles between your shoulder blades working.

To do the Dumbbell Row, place one hand on the seat of your chair and hold a dumbbell in the other. Most people find it comfortable to step back with the outside foot as shown in the picture. Keep your back straight, keep the palm of your dumbbell hand facing toward your legs and allow the dumbbell to hang toward the floor.

Keeping your back straight and your face toward the floor, raise your elbow out to the side and point it toward the ceiling, allowing your upper back to twist so that the dumbbell lightly touches your shoulder. Once the weight has touched your shoulder, gently lower it back down. One repetition should take four to five seconds.

The Dumbbell Row

Benefits: Upper Back Strength

Equipment Needed: Pair of Dumbbells, Chair

Time / Repetitions: 10-15 Repetitions

Keep your back straight.

Step back with your outside leg. This allows your torso to twist easier.

Keep your elbow straight.

Place your hand on the seat of your chair so that your fingers hang over the front edge.

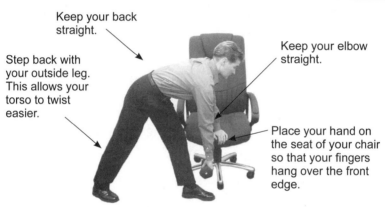

Step 1:

Point your elbow toward the ceiling while lifting the dumbbell up to your shoulder.

Keep your eyes focused on the floor.

Allow your torso to twist so that your chest faces perpendicular to the floor.

Keep your elbow straight.

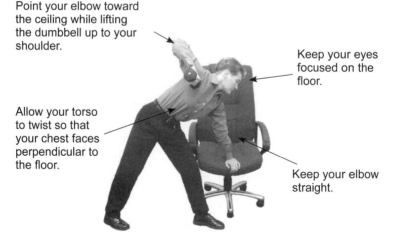

Step 2:

The Dumbbell Shrug

The Dumbbell Shrug is a great exercise for the trapezius muscle, especially the upper portion of the muscle which runs from the base of the neck, up to the base of the skull and out to the shoulders. Most people who work at desk jobs have a lot of tightness and pain in this area. The Dumbbell Shrug will help to relax the trapezius, increase circulation and decrease the "knots" in the muscle.

To do the Dumbbell Shrug, stand up straight with a dumbbell in each hand. Draw your shoulders back so that your shoulder blades squeeze together while raising your shoulders as high as you can toward your ears. Then gently let the weights back down again. Each repetition should take four to five seconds to complete.

The trapezius is considerably stronger than the rhomboid muscle. Consequently, you will be able to lift much more weight doing the Dumbbell Shrug than the Dumbbell Row. However, in order to achieve proper muscle balance in the upper back, I encourage you to use the same weight for both exercises. Here's why: in most people the trapezius is tight, inflamed and full of trigger points and already too strong in comparison to the rhomboid muscle. The goal of exercising the trapezius should not be to make it stronger but rather to improve blood flow and to decrease the amount of muscle tension. This can be accomplished by exercising the trapezius with a light weight while building strength in the rhomboids.

The Dumbbell Shrug

Benefits:	Upper Back and Neck Strength
Equipment Needed:	Pair of Dumbbells
Time / Repetitions:	10-15 Repetitions

Stand up straight and allow your shoulders to relax.

Draw your shoulders back and up as high as you can. Be sure that your shoulders don't roll forward when you lift.

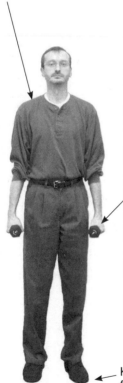

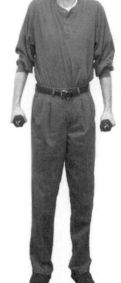

Hold a pair of dumbbells in your hands.

Keep your feet flat on the floor.

Step 1:   Step 2:

The Opening Stretch

This is a great stretch to help alleviate tension in the upper back and neck. Best of all, it only takes 30 seconds and you don't even have to get out of your chair.

To begin the Opening Stretch, scoot forward in your chair so that you are sitting comfortably on the front portion of your seat. Sit up nice and straight with both feet flat on the floor. With your upper arms hanging down to your side, bend your elbows 90 degrees and turn your palms upward so that they face toward the ceiling.

Now slowly rotate your hands outward, keeping your elbows against your torso, so that you feel a nice squeeze between the shoulder blades. Turn your feet outward as far as you can. Tip your head back slightly to remove the tension from your neck muscles, and if you'd like, close your eyes. Take three deep, slow breaths, allowing ten seconds for each breath. Just count to yourself as you breathe in "one, two, three, four, five" and back out again "six, seven, eight, nine, ten."

Many people find it beneficial to do this exercise several times during the workday, especially people who do a lot of work on a computer.

The Opening Stretch

Benefits: Upper Back and Neck Strength

Equipment Needed: Chair

Time / Repetitions: 30 Seconds

Step 1:

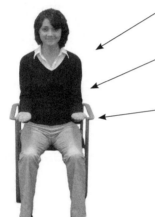

Sit up straight and slide to the front edge of your chair.

Bend your elbows 90 degrees and hold them against your side.

Turn your palms upward.

Step 2:

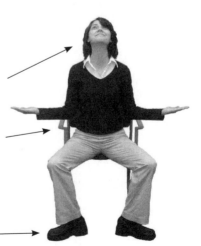

Tilt your head back and take three deep breaths.

Keeping your elbows locked to your side, rotate your hands out as far as you can.

Turn your feet outward.

The Upper Back Stretch

The Upper Back Stretch is great for improving the overall mobility and flexibility in your upper back. A very common problem with working at a desk job is that your upper back does not have the opportunity to move very much. Consequently, the joints in your spine get "sticky" and your muscles shorten. This stretch helps to keep your joints and the muscles in your upper back nice and loose.

To do the Upper Back Stretch, start by sitting up straight in your chair. Take your right hand and place it on the outside of your left knee. Twist your torso toward the left while rounding your upper back until you feel a stretch between your shoulder blades in your upper back as shown on the opposite page. Hold this position for 15 seconds, then do the Upper Back Stretch again to the opposite side.

The Upper Back Stretch

Benefits: Upper Back Flexibility

Equipment Needed: Chair

Time / Repetitions: 15 Seconds on Each Side

Twist your upper torso while rounding your back until you feel a stretch between your shoulder blades.

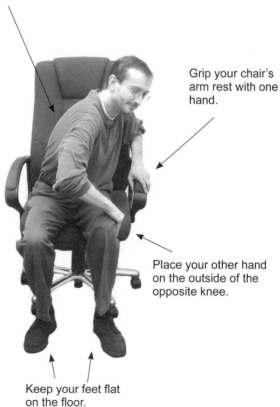

Grip your chair's arm rest with one hand.

Place your other hand on the outside of the opposite knee.

Keep your feet flat on the floor.

Neck Rolls

This simple exercise is designed to improve mobility in the neck. To do this exercise, scoot up to the front part of your seat and sit up nice and straight. Slowly let your head drop forward and let your chin drop to your chest. From that position slowly rotate your head until your right ear is resting close to your right shoulder. Then, slowly rotate your head back so that your head is tipped back as far as is comfortable. Finally, rotate your head to the left side until your left ear is resting close to your left shoulder.

It is important that you do this exercise slowly and you do not try to force your neck further than it can move comfortably. It is also important to keep your shoulders down while doing Neck Rolls. You can hold the bottom of your seat with both hands if you need help keeping your shoulders down.

Don't be surprised if you hear some crackling in your neck when you perform Neck Rolls. Usually this crackling, also called "crepitus," may go away after doing this exercise for a while, and it poses no hazard. If the crepitus does not go away, it may indicate that there is some scar tissue that has formed in the joint cartilage. Although the crackling may be annoying, it shouldn't be a cause for concern.

If you notice that your neck won't roll as well on one side as it will on the other, there may be some vertebrae that are stuck. This requires chiropractic care in order to help these vertebrae function correctly again.

Neck Rolls

Benefits:	Neck Mobility
Equipment Needed:	Chair
Time / Repetitions:	15 Rotations in Each Direction

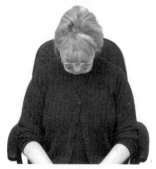

Step 1:

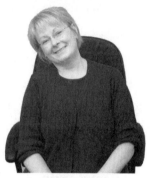

Step 2:

When doing Neck Rolls, it is important to do three things in order to properly stretch the muscles of the neck: 1) keep your shoulders perfectly level, 2) keep your face oriented forward, and 3) roll your head slowly. It should take 30 seconds to make one complete revolution.

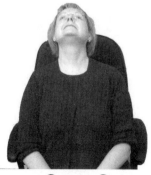

Step 3:

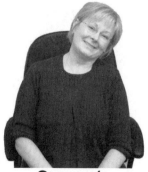

Step 4:

The Chair Neck Stretch

The Chair Neck Stretch can be used to decrease the tightness of the trapezius and levator scapulae, as well as the scalene muscles. To do the Chair Neck Stretch, scoot up to the front edge of your chair and sit up straight. With your right hand, grasp the bottom of the seat of your chair. Reach over the top of your head with your left hand and place it on the right side of your head. Gently lean toward the left while tipping your head to the left until you feel a good stretch in the neck and shoulder muscles. Hold this stretch for 30-45 seconds, then switch sides.

You can vary the muscles stretched by placing your hand on different parts of your chair seat and leaning your head at different angles. To stretch primarily your trapezius and levator scapulae, grip your seat just behind your hip and tilt your head slightly forward and to the side. To stretch primarily your scalenes, grip your seat at about your mid-thigh and tilt your head slightly backward and to the side. Remember that the muscles of the neck are small and somewhat fragile, so stretch gently and hold without bouncing.

The Chair Neck Stretch

Benefits: Neck Mobility

Equipment Needed: Chair

Time / Repetitions: 30-40 Seconds on Each Side

Place your hand on the side of your head and gently pull to increase the stretch on your neck muscles.

Tilt your head to the side until you feel a stretch.

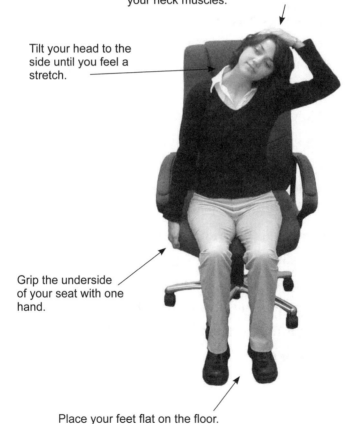

Grip the underside of your seat with one hand.

Place your feet flat on the floor.

The Wall Posture

This simple exercise is designed to directly counteract the unhealthy neck and upper back posture found in people who work at desk jobs; namely, the head being carried too far forward and the hunching of the upper back.

To do this exercise, simply stand up against a wall, making sure that your heels, pelvis, shoulders and the back of your head are all touching the wall. Make sure that your head stays level and that you glide your head backward, rather than tilting your head back in order to touch the wall with your head. This will require you to pull your chin down toward your chest a bit.

Once you have successfully positioned yourself into this Wall Posture, slowly step away from the wall and go about your business while holding the posture as long as possible. If you have done this correctly, it will probably feel somewhat unusual to walk around like this. But don't worry, you don't look as funny as you feel. As a matter of fact, to everyone else, you probably look better. People with good posture look better than those with bad posture.

It is important that you try to hold this posture while you go back about your business in order to retrain your body mechanics. For this reason, most people find it necessary to do this exercise several times throughout the day as a checkup on their posture.

The Wall Posture

Benefits: Neck and Upper Back Posture

Equipment Needed: Wall

Time / Repetitions: Maintain as Long as Possible

Stand up against a wall so that your shoulders, hips and heels are all touching the wall.

Keeping your head level, draw your neck back until the back of your head touches the wall.

Step away from the wall while maintaining this new head posture. Keep this head posture as long as you can while you work.

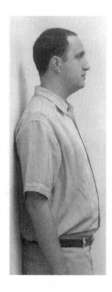

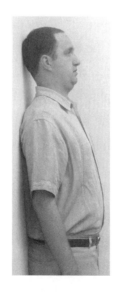

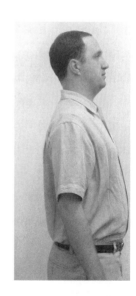

Step 1:   Step 2:   Step 3:

Stiff-Leg Deadlifts

With the exception of abdominal muscle strengthening, the Stiff-Leg Deadlift is the single-most important exercise to strengthen and recoordinate all of the muscles of the low back and pelvis. To do this exercise, you will want to start by standing up straight with your feet about shoulder width apart, a pair of dumbbells in your hands and your knees bent slightly — about 10-15 degrees. The object is to bend forward at the hips, allowing the dumbbells to drop just below the knees and then to straighten back up again, all the while keeping your head up, your back straight, and your knees bent slightly.

It is very important when bending at the hips that you do not cheat and bend at the waist. If you do this exercise correctly, you should feel most of the exercise in your hamstrings rather than in your low back. If you feel it mostly in your low back, it means that you are not pushing your hips back far enough and that you are bending at the waist. Many people find it helpful to imagine that they are carefully sitting down on a chair behind them while keeping their back straight.

You will want each repetition of lowering the weights down and lifting them back up to take approximately six to eight seconds. One other thing about the Stiff-Leg Deadlifts: since you are working large muscles, you will want to use dumbbells that are heavy enough to challenge the muscles; 15-25 pound dumbbells are probably a good place to start.

Stiff-Leg Deadlifts

Benefits: Low Back Strength and Coordination

Equipment Needed: Pair of Dumbbells

Time / Repetitions: 10-15 Repetitions

Draw your shoulders back.

Bend forward at the hips. You should feel a stretch in the back of your legs.

Keep your back straight. Don't bend at the waist.

Hold a pair of dumbbells in your hands.

Bend your knees slightly.

Keep your chin up.

Step 1:

Allow weights to drop below your knees.

Step 2:

Pelvic Tilts

Pelvic Tilts are one of the easiest exercises to help increase abdominal strength. To do this exercise, stand up straight and place your hands on your hips. Exhale completely while contracting your abdominal muscles and tilting your pelvis as shown in the picture on the opposite page. Hold this position for three seconds, then inhale and allow your body to return to the starting position. Each repetition should take approximately three to five seconds.

Depending on the condition of your body when you begin doing Pelvic Tilts, you may feel your abdominals getting a good workout from this exercise, but don't be discouraged if you do not feel this at first.

You can make this exercise even more intense by drawing your abdomen in as far as you can after you completely exhale. You should feel a contraction in your oblique muscles just to the side of your abdominals. This extra contraction of the obliques helps to flatten the belly.

Pelvic Tilts

Benefits: Abdominal Strength

Equipment Needed: None

Time / Repetitions: As Many as Possible

Step 1:   Step 2:

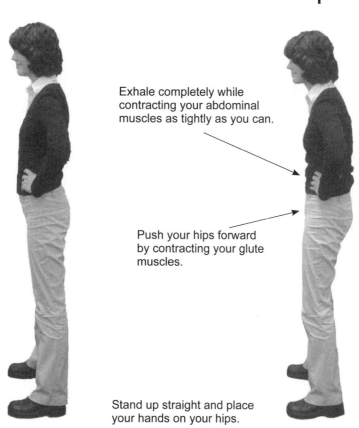

Exhale completely while contracting your abdominal muscles as tightly as you can.

Push your hips forward by contracting your glute muscles.

Stand up straight and place your hands on your hips.

Chair Crunches

Chair Crunches are designed to help increase abdominal strength while improving balance and coordination. To do this exercise, scoot forward in the seat of your chair so that your buttocks rest on the front edge of the seat but the backs of your legs are not touching the chair. Keeping your back straight, lean back slightly and grip the armrests of your chair with both hands. Using your abdominal muscles, raise your knees as far toward your chest as you can. Hold this position for one second and then slowly lower your knees back down. Each repetition should take approximately three to four seconds.

You can decrease the difficulty of this exercise by keeping your knees bent so that your feet stay close to your body. The more you straighten your legs, the more difficult this exercise becomes.

Depending on the condition of your body when you begin doing Chair Crunches, you may feel your abdominals getting a good workout from this exercise, but don't be discouraged if you do not feel this at first. Initially, you may feel it more in your low back or even legs. This is common when the abdominal muscles have lost their natural coordination. Just keep at it and soon your abdominal muscles will come around.

Chair Crunches

Benefits: Abdominal Strength

Equipment Needed: Chair

Time / Repetitions: As Many as Possible Without Pain

Step 1:

Grip your armrests for support.

Scoot up to the front edge of your chair.

Straighten your legs out in front of you so that your heels rest on the floor.

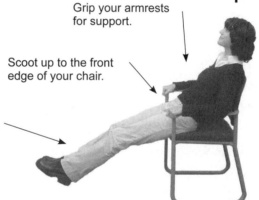

Draw your knees up as close to your chest as you can.

Note: You can increase the intensity of this exercise by not allowing your heels to touch the floor each time you straighten your legs.

Step 2:

The Cobra Stretch

The Cobra Stretch is great for improving the flexibility of the abdominal and psoas muscles as well as increasing mobility in the low back. When doing this exercise, be sure that your chair is pushed up against a wall so that it doesn't move away from you. To do the Cobra Stretch, stand facing your chair, with your feet shoulder width apart and about 24"-36" away from the edge of your chair. Lean forward and grip the center of your armrests. Keeping your arms straight, allow your pelvis to drop toward the seat of your chair and lift your chin toward the ceiling. You should feel a considerable stretch in the abdominals when you do this stretch correctly.

You can adjust the intensity of the stretch by how far you place your feet from your chair. The farther away your feet are, the more intense the stretch will be on your abdominal muscles.

Depending on the strength of your upper body, you may find it difficult to support your weight with your arms for very long. If this happens, you can step forward with your feet slightly to decrease the weight supported by the arms and make sure that you keep your elbows straight. After a few weeks of doing this stretch, your arms will become stronger and it will be easier to support yourself.

Discontinue doing this stretch if you feel pain in your low back and just stick with the other low back exercises and stretches for a couple of weeks before trying this stretch again. As your back becomes healthier, you should be able to do this stretch without experiencing back pain.

The Cobra Stretch

Benefits: Flexibility in the Low Back

Equipment Needed: Chair

Time / Repetitions: 30-45 Seconds

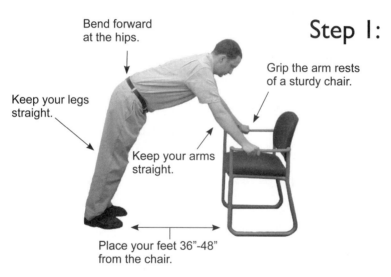

Bend forward at the hips.

Step 1:

Grip the arm rests of a sturdy chair.

Keep your legs straight.

Keep your arms straight.

Place your feet 36"-48" from the chair.

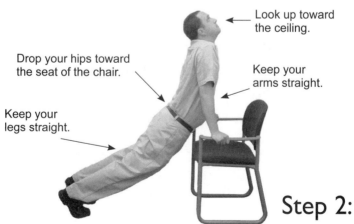

Look up toward the ceiling.

Drop your hips toward the seat of the chair.

Keep your arms straight.

Keep your legs straight.

Step 2:

The Chair Low Back Stretch

This stretch is a quick way to reduce tension in the low back and is perfect for a mini-break during the day. To do this stretch, scoot forward to the front part of your seat and straighten your legs. Allowing your spine to bend forward, reach your hands as far down the front of your legs as possible and allow your head to drop toward your thighs. Take slow, deep breaths for 30-45 seconds, then sit back up again.

If you have a difficult time getting your low back to bend forward, which many people do, it could be for a couple of reasons. The first is that if your hamstring muscles are too tight, they will hold your pelvis in place and not allow it to roll forward. If your pelvis cannot roll forward, your low back will not be able to bend as far forward. If this is the case with you, doing hamstring stretches will help.

The other reason why you may not be able roll your back forward is that the joints in your low back are stuck and are not allowing the vertebrae to move correctly. This is very common among people who work at desk jobs. The only way to get the joints in the low back moving correctly again is through chiropractic care. If this stretch is difficult for you, it is a good idea to have your low back checked out by a chiropractor.

The Chair Low Back Stretch

Benefits: Decrease Tension in the Low Back

Equipment Needed: Chair

Time / Repetitions: 30-45 Seconds

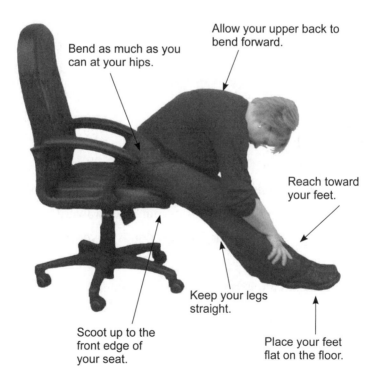

Allow your upper back to bend forward.

Bend as much as you can at your hips.

Reach toward your feet.

Scoot up to the front edge of your seat.

Keep your legs straight.

Place your feet flat on the floor.

The Glute Medius Stretch

The Glute Medius Stretch is very effective in reducing the stress in the hip and buttock area. To do this stretch, scoot up to the front part of your seat and rest the ankle of one leg on the thigh of the other. Sit up nice and straight and place both hands around the knee of your topmost leg, interlacing your fingers. Using a gentle pull, draw your knee up to the opposite shoulder and hold the position for 30-45 seconds. Then switch legs and do the same stretch to the other leg. If you do this stretch correctly, you should feel a good stretch in the buttock.

This stretch is very important for people who sit a lot at work because the muscles in the buttocks and pelvis become very tight. This tightness contributes to pain and loss of flexibility in the low back.

If you find that you don't have enough flexibility to cross your legs as pictured, you can start by gripping one knee with both of your hands and pulling your knee toward your chest and holding the stretch for 30-45 seconds. Over time, the glute medius and piriformis muscles will relax and allow you to perform the stretch as shown.

The Glute Medius Stretch

Benefits: Pelvis and Hip Flexibility

Equipment Needed: Chair

Time / Repetitions: 30-45 Seconds on Each Side

Step 1:

Step 2:

Sit up straight in your chair.

Cross one leg over the other and grab your knee with both hands.

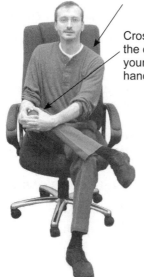
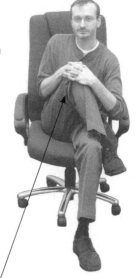

Keeping your back straight, pull your knee up as high up toward the opposite shoulder as you can. Hold the stretch for 30-45 seconds.

The Psoas Stretch

A tight psoas muscle is one of the biggest contributors to the low back pain experienced by most people who sit at work. This stretch is designed to decrease the tension in the psoas muscle and improve the mobility and flexibility in the low back. To do this stretch, start with both feet together, your back straight and one of your hands resting on your chair or a wall for balance. Take a large step back with one of your legs as shown in the picture on the opposite page. Keeping your back leg straight and allowing your front leg to bend at the knee, push the hip of your back leg forward until you feel a stretch in the upper inside front part of the thigh. Hold this stretch for 30-45 seconds, then switch legs.

The key to doing this stretch is keeping the hips in the correct position. If you do not feel a stretch in the right place, it is likely that you are allowing your hips to turn to the side and are not keeping them facing the front. The other thing that could be happening is that you may be trying to keep your back foot flat on the floor. In order for the back leg to have enough mobility to stretch the psoas muscle, it will be necessary to raise your heel.

If you have good balance, you can increase the intensity of the stretch by raising your hands above your head and tipping your upper body backwards slightly while looking at the ceiling. This offers you the added benefit of stretching the abdominal muscles at the same time.

The Psoas Stretch

Benefits: Low Back and Pelvis Flexibility

Equipment Needed: None

Time / Repetitions: 30-45 Seconds on Each Side

Stand up straight and place your hands on your hips.

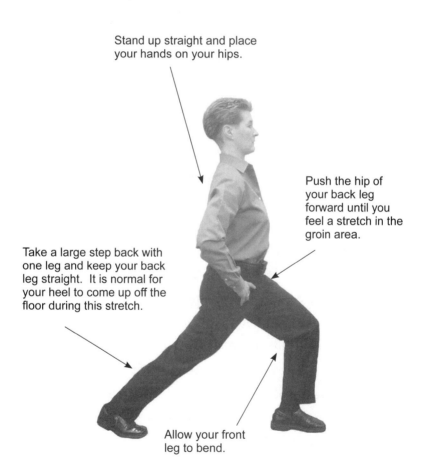

Push the hip of your back leg forward until you feel a stretch in the groin area.

Take a large step back with one leg and keep your back leg straight. It is normal for your heel to come up off the floor during this stretch.

Allow your front leg to bend.

The Lunge

You can do Lunges with or without weights depending on your physical condition. If you have not done Lunges before, I suggest that you start without weights. To do the Lunge, start with your feet together and one hand resting on the back of a chair for balance. Step back with one leg so that your legs are about 60 degrees apart. Keeping your back straight, allow your knees to bend until you touch the floor with the knee of your back leg, then straighten your legs again. Repeat this exercise 10-15 times for each leg.

If you have knee problems, you may have to modify the Lunge somewhat to make it easier on your knees. One way of doing this is to place a phone book or two on the floor in front of your back leg so that your back knee only drops to within six inches from the floor. If this is still too stressful for your knees, just go down as far as you can. The further down you can go, the better, as long as it doesn't strain your knees.

This is a great exercise to improve the strength and flexibility in the quadriceps and glute muscles as well as to improve your overall coordination and sense of balance. After doing Lunges for a while, you will notice that it is easier to climb stairs, easier to squat down to grab something off of the floor, and that there will be less soreness in your buttocks and legs from prolonged sitting.

The Lunge

Benefits: Quadriceps and Glute Strength

Equipment Needed: Chair

Time / Repetitions: 10-15 Repetitions for Each Leg

Step 1:

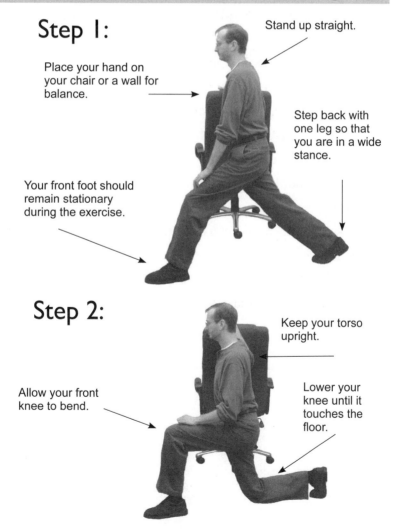

Stand up straight.

Place your hand on your chair or a wall for balance.

Step back with one leg so that you are in a wide stance.

Your front foot should remain stationary during the exercise.

Step 2:

Keep your torso upright.

Allow your front knee to bend.

Lower your knee until it touches the floor.

Calf Raises

Calf Raises are great for improving the strength and flexibility of your calf muscles. To do Calf Raises you will need a phone book or a stair step. Begin by placing the ball of your foot on the edge of the step or phone book so that your heel hangs freely in the air. Slowly lower your heel as far as you can, then raise your heel up as high as you can and hold this for one second. You will probably have to place your hand on the back of your chair or on a wall to maintain your balance when doing this exercise. Repeat this exercise 20-30 times.

One of the problems with a desk job is that most people begin to suffer the effects from decreased circulation in the legs. The veins in your legs require the exercise of the leg muscles in order to move your blood back to your heart effectively. When this does not happen, you can develop varicose and spider veins as well as swelling around the ankles.

The leg exercises in this section will go a long way to counteracting the decreased circulation in the legs, which is associated with sitting.

Calf Raises

Benefits: Calf Strength

Equipment Needed: Stair Step or Phone Book

Time / Repetitions: 20-30 Repetitions

Note: When doing Calf Raises, you will want to place your hand on a chair or a wall to help maintain your balance.

Place the ball of your foot at the edge of the phone book, allowing your heels to hang over the edge. ——————————→

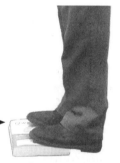

Step 1:

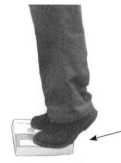

Lift your heels up as high as you can and hold them in this position for one second before lowering them back to the floor.

Step 2:

As an alternative, you can do this exercise on a stair step or any other object that is at least two inches high. To make this exercise a bit more challenging, try doing this exercise using only one leg at a time.

The Quadriceps Stretch

The Quadriceps Stretch is a great way to reduce the tension and improve the flexibility in the front of the thigh. To do the Quadriceps Stretch, start by standing next to chair or a wall and placing your hand on it for balance. Raise one foot backwards by bending your knee and grasping the foot with your free hand. Gently pull your leg back and press your foot against your buttock until you feel a stretch in the front part of your thigh. Hold this position for 30-45 seconds, then slowly release your hand from your foot and allow your foot to drop back to the floor. Repeat this stretch on the opposite leg.

Since the quadriceps are such big muscle groups, you will notice an immediate decrease in your overall tension level just by doing this stretch. This maneuver along with the next two stretches for the hamstrings and the calves should be done at least once a day for maximum benefit. I recommend doing each of these stretches twice per day, once early and once in the later part of the day.

The Quadriceps Stretch

Benefits: Quadriceps Flexibility

Equipment Needed: None

Time / Repetitions: 30-45 Seconds on Each Side

Stand up nice and straight and place your hand on a chair or a wall for balance.

Do not lean forward during the stretch.

Bend your knee and grab your foot with your hand.

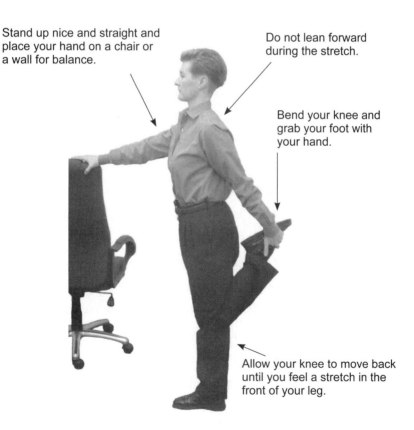

Allow your knee to move back until you feel a stretch in the front of your leg.

The Triangle Stretch

The Triangle Stretch is great for improving the flexibility of the hamstrings and adductors. To do this stretch, start by facing your chair; place both hands on the arm rests and place your feet as far apart as you comfortably can. Slowly bend at the hips so that your pelvis drops back behind your feet and your body drops toward the seat of your chair. You should feel a good stretch in your hamstrings, as well as in the inside part of your upper leg. Hold this stretch for 30-45 seconds without bouncing.

If you don't feel a stretch in the back of your legs, you may be doing one of three things incorrectly. First, you may have your feet too far away from the chair; try moving your feet a little closer. Second, you may not have your feet spread far enough; try moving them a little farther apart. Third, you may be bending at the waist instead of at the hips; try bending more at the hips as in the Stiff-Leg Deadlifts.

The Triangle Stretch is a must for people with desk jobs, as prolonged sitting causes the hamstrings to tighten up. If you do this stretch regularly, you will notice an improvement in your flexibility, you will be more comfortable when you have to sit for long periods, and it will even decrease the stress on your low back, helping to reduce back pain.

The Triangle Stretch

Benefits:	Hamstrings and Adductor Flexibility
Equipment Needed:	Chair
Time / Repetitions:	30-45 Seconds

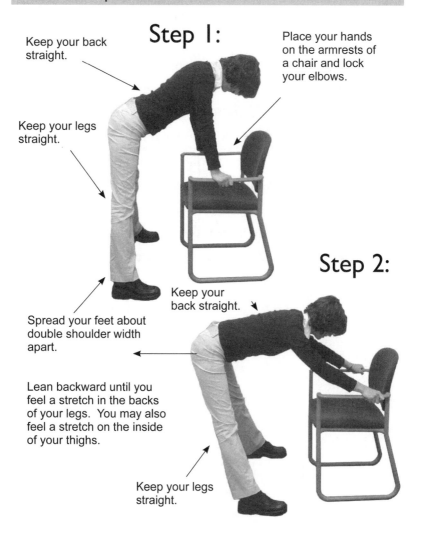

Step 1:

Keep your back straight.

Place your hands on the armrests of a chair and lock your elbows.

Keep your legs straight.

Spread your feet about double shoulder width apart.

Step 2:

Keep your back straight.

Lean backward until you feel a stretch in the backs of your legs. You may also feel a stretch on the inside of your thighs.

Keep your legs straight.

The Calf Stretch

The Calf Stretch is one of three important stretches, along with the Triangle Stretch and the Quadriceps Stretch, that will keep your legs flexible and relaxed during a long day at work. To do this stretch, start by facing a wall approximately an arm's length away. Place both hands on the wall and take a big step back with one of your legs, allowing the leg closest to the wall to bend at the knee. Gently allow your back heel to drop toward the floor until you feel a stretch in your calf muscles. Hold this stretch for 30-45 seconds without bouncing, then switch legs.

As you read in the Calf Raises exercise description, the calf muscles are not only responsible for walking, but they also help with pumping blood back to the heart. When the calf muscles, and to some degree the hamstrings, are chronically tight and don't get enough exercise, blood tends to pool in the lower legs and can lead to painful varicose veins and swelling in the ankles.

The Calf Stretch

Benefits:	Calf Flexibility
Equipment Needed:	Wall
Time / Repetitions:	30-45 Seconds on Each Side

Place your hands against a wall.

Keep your back straight.

Place the leg you are going to stretch behind you as far as you can.

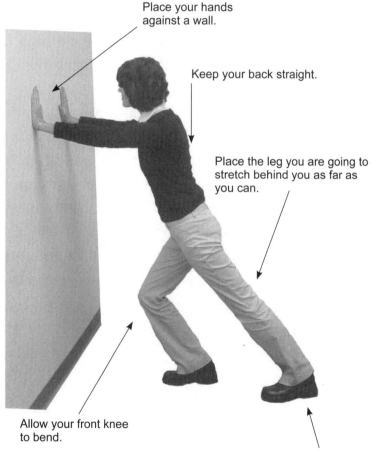

Allow your front knee to bend.

Slowly drop your heel to the floor so that you feel a stretch in your calf muscles.

Desk Push-Ups

Desk Push-Ups are a great way to improve the strength of the pec major muscles. To do this exercise, start by placing both hands on the edge of your desk. Step back so that your body is angled about 45 degrees from the floor and hold your body away from your desk with your arms straight. Bend your elbows and lower your body all the way down until your chest touches the front edge of the desk, then straighten your arms again to raise your body back up. Repeat this exercise for a total of 10-20 repetitions.

If you haven't done much strength training, this exercise may seem very difficult or impossible at first. If you are unable to do at least ten push-ups where you touch your chest to your desk, start out by only going down halfway. It is important to do at least ten repetitions in order to work the muscle enough to increase strength. As you become stronger, you will be able to drop your body closer and closer to your desk. One other thing that you can do if you find this exercise too challenging at first is to place your feet closer to your desk. The closer your feet are to your desk, the easier this exercise will be, at least to a point. You can modify this exercise as you need as long as you are able to do the exercise comfortably.

Desk Push-Ups

Benefits: Pec Major Strength

Equipment Needed: Desk

Time / Repetitions: 10-20 Repetitions

Keep your back straight.

Place your feet back far enough so that your body makes a 45 degree angle to the floor.

Place your hands on the edge of your desk.

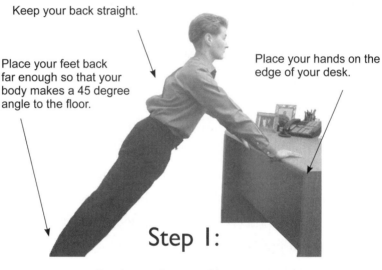

Step 1:

Bend your elbows and lower your chest to your desk, then push yourself back up.

Keep your back straight.

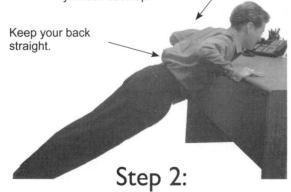

Step 2:

The Stick-Em Up Stretch

The Stick-Em Up Stretch is great for decreasing the tension of the pec minor muscle, allowing the shoulders to roll back to a healthier posture and decreasing any tingling and numbness in the arms that may be present. This stretch is called the Stick-Em Up stretch because you start by assuming the posture often seen in old Western movies when the villain says "Stick 'em up!" Your upper arms should be parallel to the floor, with your elbows bent 90 degrees so that your hands are raised above your head with your palms facing forward. With your arms in that position, step into a doorway so that your forearms rest against the door frame. Be sure that your feet are centered within the doorway. Gently push your hips forward until you feel a stretch in your upper chest and shoulders. Hold this position without bouncing for 30-45 seconds, then step away from the doorway and allow your hands to drop to your side.

It is important that this stretch be done on a daily basis. When the pec minor is tight, it causes one of the major components of the Foreward Head Posture—the dreaded forward shoulders and the resultant hunching of the upper back.

The Stick-Em Up Stretch

Benefits: Pec Minor Flexibility

Equipment Needed: Doorway

Time / Repetitions: 30-45 Seconds

Face your palms forward.

Bend your elbows 90 degrees and raise your upper arms so that they are parallel to the floor.

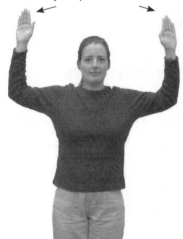

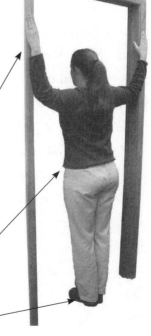

Place your forearms against a door frame.

Stand up straight and gently lean forward until you feel a stretch in your upper pecs. Hold this position for 30-45 seconds.

Bring your feet into the doorway so that you are not bending forward.

Dumbbell Curls

The Dumbbell Curl is the simplest, most effective way to improve the strength in the biceps muscle. To do this exercise, start by standing up straight and holding one dumbbell in each hand; palms facing forward. Using only the muscles in your arm, lift the weight up to your shoulder by bending your elbow. Once you raise the weight as far as you can, gently lower it back down again. One entire repetition should take three to four seconds.

It is important when doing this exercise to keep your elbows locked to your side and not move them forward or backward—that's cheating. The other important thing is to keep your body from swaying back when you raise the dumbbell—that's also cheating. My favorite way to do this exercise is to alternate hands so that while I am raising a dumbbell with one hand, I am lowering the dumbbell in the other. But you may prefer to only exercise one arm at a time. Either way is okay as long as you do 10-15 repetitions with each arm. As with the other exercises which utilize weights, if you are able to do 16 repetitions, you need to increase the weight you are lifting. If you are unable to do ten repetitions, you will need to decrease the weight you are using.

This exercise is particularly effective in reducing the tightness in your biceps if you immediately follow it up with the Biceps Door Stretch.

Dumbbell Curls

Benefits: Biceps Strength

Equipment Needed: Pair of Dumbbells

Time / Repetitions: 10-15 Repetitions for Each Arm

Keep your back straight.

Raise the dumbbell up to your shoulder, then lower it back down again.

Hold your elbows tight to your side.

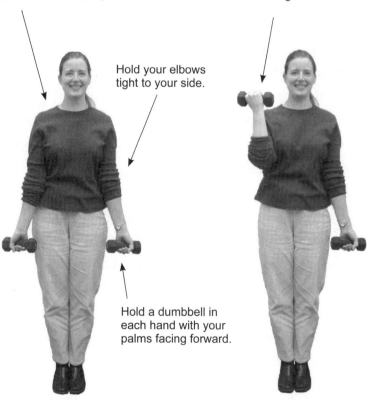

Hold a dumbbell in each hand with your palms facing forward.

Step 1:

Step 2:

Chair Dips

This exercise does wonders for the strength of the triceps muscle and, to a lesser degree, the muscles in the front of the shoulder. To do this exercise, start by leaning against the edge of your chair, place your hands on either side and grip the arms of your chair. Move your hips about 12"-18" away from the edge of the chair by moving your feet forward, while keeping your arms straight and your hands gripping the arms of the chair. Keeping your back straight and your head up, lower your hips as far as you can toward the floor by bending your elbows, then straighten your arms to lift yourself up again. Repeat this exercise for a total of 10-15 repetitions.

Depending on your condition, you may find this exercise to be very difficult. Don't worry if you cannot do ten repetitions, or even five repetitions for that matter, when you first try this exercise. If you just keep doing Chair Dips, you will gradually become stronger and they will become easier.

One trick that works well when you cannot do ten repetitions of a particular exercise is to break up the routine into smaller chunks. You may want to do five repetitions, take a short break, then do five more. You can even break it into two-repetition chunks if you have to, and do two repetitions five times throughout the day.

Chair Dips

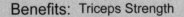

Benefits: Triceps Strength

Equipment Needed: Chair

Time / Repetitions: 10-15 Repetitions

Step 1:

Look straight ahead.

Place your feet out in front of you far enough so that there is 12"-18" of space between your hips and the chair seat.

Place your hands either on the arm rests or the seat of a stable chair.

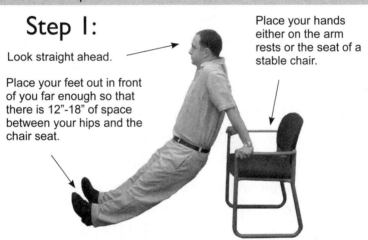

Step 2:

Look straight ahead.

Keep your legs straight.

Lower your hips toward the floor by bending your elbows, then push yourself back up again.

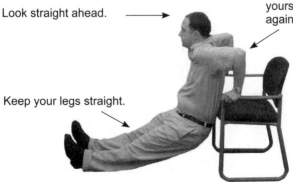

The Overhead Press

The Overhead Press is a great overall exercise to improve the strength in the triceps and shoulders. Begin by grasping a pair of dumbbells and raising them up to your shoulders, palms facing forward as shown in the picture on the opposite page. Raise the weights above your head by straightening your arms and bring the weights together so that they touch. Then gently lower the weights back down to the level of your shoulders. Repeat for a total of 10-15 repetitions.

If you have never done this exercise before, your arms may feel fairly wobbly and uncoordinated. This is normal and will go away after a couple of weeks of doing the exercise. It is also common for people who have not done this exercise before to feel like their muscles are not getting a very good workout. This happens because you are asking your muscles to work in a way that they are not used to, so they will be a bit uncoordinated. Just keep doing the exercise and you will eventually feel your muscles begin to get a good workout.

It is important when doing the Overhead Press that two basic safety rules are followed. The first is that you should not use a weight that is too heavy for you. If you cannot do ten repetitions, you need to use a lighter weight. The second is that you should not use dumbbells that have removable plates. Instead, use solid-cast, one-piece dumbbells that cannot come apart and cause injury when they are raised above your head.

The Overhead Press

Benefits: Shoulder and Triceps Strength

Equipment Needed: Pair of Dumbbells

Time / Repetitions: 10-15 Repetitions

Hold a dumbbell in each hand with your palms facing forward.

Raise the dumbbells above your head as high as you can until they gently touch.

Sit up straight.

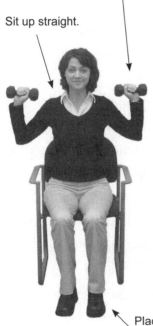

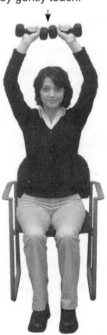

Place your feet flat on the floor.

Step 1:

Step 2:

The Biceps Door Stretch

The Biceps Door Stretch is a very effective way to decrease the tightness in the biceps muscles. To do this stretch, begin by gripping the frame of a door so that your thumb points toward the floor as shown in the picture on the opposite page. Slide your hand up to just below the level of your shoulder. Turn your body so that your arm is directly behind you and your shoulders are parallel to the wall. Gently push your pelvis forward until you feel a stretch in your upper arm. Hold the stretch for 30-45 seconds, then switch arms and do the same. When you switch arms, you will have to move to the other side of the door frame.

This stretch can be a bit tricky. If you do not feel a stretch in your arm, you are probably doing one of two things incorrectly. The first and most common mistake that most people make is that their shoulders are not parallel to the wall where the door is located. Make sure that your shoulders are lined up with the wall and not in a straight line with your arm. The second mistake is not raising your hand high enough behind you. This is easily corrected by simply sliding your hand up further. As long as your shoulders are square with the wall, you will eventually reach a point where you feel a stretch in your biceps muscle.

You can make this stretch even more effective by performing it immediately following your Dumbbell Curls when your muscles are nice and warm.

The Biceps Door Stretch

Benefits: Biceps Flexibility

Equipment Needed: Doorway

Time / Repetitions: 30-45 Seconds on Each Side

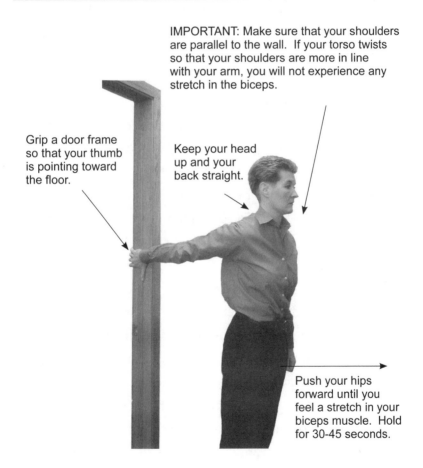

IMPORTANT: Make sure that your shoulders are parallel to the wall. If your torso twists so that your shoulders are more in line with your arm, you will not experience any stretch in the biceps.

Grip a door frame so that your thumb is pointing toward the floor.

Keep your head up and your back straight.

Push your hips forward until you feel a stretch in your biceps muscle. Hold for 30-45 seconds.

The Wrist Stretch

The Wrist Stretch is designed to decrease the tension in your forearms and wrists. To do this stretch straighten out one of your arms and allow your wrist to relax. Take your other hand and gently pull your wrist into further flexion as shown in Step 1 in the picture on the opposite page. Hold this stretch for 30-45 seconds, then switch directions and pull your hand upwards to stretch the forearm flexors. Hold this stretch for 30-45 seconds, then switch hands.

To get the most out of this stretch, it is best to do it at least twice per day; three times would be even better. Be careful not to pull too hard on your hand and over-stretch the muscles in your forearms. Those muscles are fairly small and can be strained easily.

If you suffer from Carpal Tunnel Syndrome, this stretch may cause some tingling in your hands. Minor tingling is probably not a major concern and should improve after a few days of doing this stretch. However, if the pain or tingling in your hands is moderate to severe, only do the Wrist Stretch to the point where the pain begins, then back off a bit.

When you experience tingling in your hands by doing the Wrist Stretch, it indicates that the median nerve which runs through the center of your wrist is being pinched. You don't want to pinch it too much or you may cause the nerve to become irritated or injured. So remember, a little tingling is okay when doing the Wrist Stretch, but a lot of tingling or pain is a sign that you are overdoing it a bit.

The Wrist Stretch

Benefits:	Wrist and Forearm Flexibility
Equipment Needed:	None
Time / Repetitions:	30-45 Seconds

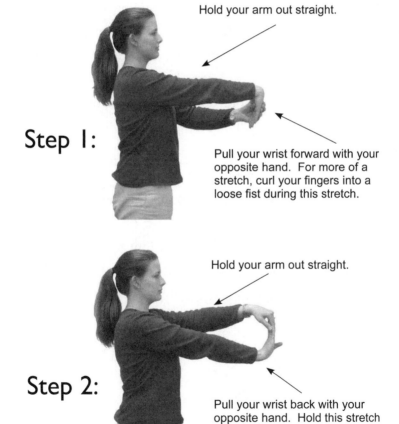

Hold your arm out straight.

Step 1:

Pull your wrist forward with your opposite hand. For more of a stretch, curl your fingers into a loose fist during this stretch.

Hold your arm out straight.

Step 2:

Pull your wrist back with your opposite hand. Hold this stretch for 30-45 seconds.

The Prayer Stretch

This stretch is great for decreasing the tension in your hands, fingers, and wrists. To do the Prayer Stretch, start by spreading your fingers apart a little and touching the fingertips of your two hands together, keeping your fingers straight. Gently push your palms toward each other while lowering your hands just enough to keep your palms from touching, as shown in the picture on the opposite page. At this point, you should feel a stretch in your hands and wrists. Holding the separation between your palms, rotate your wrists so that at one extreme your thumb is level with your stomach and at the other extreme your little finger touches your belt line, as shown in the pictures on the opposite page.

This stretch really needs to be done gently and often. The muscles and connective tissues in your hands, fingers, and wrists are very small and prone to strain, so go for a good stretch, but don't overdo it. Since people with desk jobs tend to hold their hands in a semi-closed position most of the day, this stretch will really help re-establish normal flexibility.

The Prayer Stretch

Benefits: Hand and Wrist Flexibility

Equipment Needed: None

Time / Repetitions: 30-45 Seconds

Touch your fingertips together and point your fingers toward the ceiling.

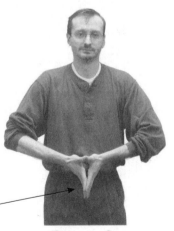

Gently press your hands together without allowing your palms to touch, until you feel a stretch. Hold for 30-45 seconds.

Step 1:

Keeping the pressure on your fingertips, rotate your wrists so that your fingers point toward the floor. Hold for an additional 20-30 seconds.

Step 2:

Recommended Resources

For training, always work with a certified professional. Some of the best trainers are certified through these organizations:

- *IDEA Health & Fitness Association*
- *National Strength and Conditioning Association (NSCA)*
- *National Academy of Sports Medicine (NASM)*
- *American College of Sports Medicine (ACSM)*

11

Nutrition

T hink about this for a moment: every single cell in your body is made up from the material that you put into your mouth. The old saying "garbage in, garbage out" is especially true when it comes to nutrition. Just as a house cannot be strong if it is made with poor materials, your body cannot be healthy and strong if you don't feed it properly. Unfortunately, too many people consume an endless stream of pizza, soft drinks, fast foods, and processed sugar; and then they wonder why there is such an epidemic of obesity, diabetes, heart disease and cancer in our culture. In order for there to be more people less sick, it is absolutely necessary to make good nutrition a part of our daily routine.

Who doesn't already know that the foods you choose to eat and how much of them you eat will positively or negatively affect your health? Why do so many people literally eat themselves to death? The truth is that why you eat is more important than what

you eat. Most people these days don't simply eat when they are
hungry and stop when they are full. Millions of people use food
as an emotional comfort or as an escape. Some people become
obese to justify or reinforce their low opinions of themselves;
others overeat due to depression. These are the deeper issues
that must be faced in order to make lasting, positive changes in
our diet.

Food is not simply an energy source for the body. Each
piece of food you put into your mouth contains hundreds or
thousands of individual chemicals that influence a wide range of
functions in your body, including your metabolic rate, immune
function, emotional state, and your body weight. It is important
to understand how carbohydrates, proteins, and fats influence
your body's biochemistry so that you can make informed choices
about the foods you eat. Once you understand some simple
ideas about food, you can use this knowledge to lose weight and
improve your overall health. In this chapter, you will learn how
your body uses the three basic types of food—carbohydrates,
fats, and proteins. You will also learn about certain vitamins and
minerals that can be critical to your well-being.

Carbohydrates

Carbohydrates are the main fuel source that your body uses
to think, run, walk, breathe, or do just about anything else. Next
to water, carbohydrates are the most consumed nutrients in the
world. There are three types of carbohydrates that you consume
every day: sugars, complex carbohydrates, and fiber.

In order for the body to use the sugars and starches in food, it must first break them down to a form that can be used by your body's cells. The first step of the digestion processes occurs in your mouth by an enzyme called salivary amylase. This enzyme begins the process of breaking down starches into simple sugars. Once food reaches your stomach, the digestion of carbohydrates stops. It begins again once your food leaves the stomach and enters the small intestine.

The main purpose of the digestion process is to convert the carbohydrates you consume into a simple sugar called glucose. Glucose is the form of carbohydrate that is the primary fuel source for the brain, central nervous system, and nearly every other cell in your body.

To ensure a readily available supply of glucose, the body stores it in the muscle and liver in a form called glycogen. Glycogen is then converted back to glucose any time your blood glucose level drops too low. If your body uses up all its glycogen, it will start breaking down muscle in order to provide your vital organs with the glucose they need to function.

The two major hormones that help regulate the level of glucose in your blood are insulin and glucagon. Insulin is a hormone that is released when your blood glucose levels rise, as typically occurs after you consume food containing carbohydrate. The function of insulin is to signal the liver and muscle cells to remove the excess glucose from the blood and store it as glycogen.

Glucagon has the opposite effect. When your blood glucose levels become too low, glucagon will signal the muscle and liver to convert glycogen back to glucose and release it into the blood stream. The balance of these two hormones helps to keep blood glucose levels within a fairly narrow range.

There are some instances when the body is unable to maintain healthy blood glucose levels. The most common condition is called diabetes and is caused by a loss of normal insulin function. Those with diabetes have an abnormally high blood glucose level. A much rarer condition called primary hypoglycemia describes blood glucose levels which are abnormally low.

Not all carbohydrates have the same effect on blood glucose levels. Starches are much larger molecules than sugars and therefore take longer to break down and enter the blood stream. Sugars, on the other hand, are simple molecules that can quickly be converted into glucose and enter the blood. Sugars will tend to create a sharp spike in blood glucose levels, whereas starches will tend to cause a much more gradual increase.

The measure of a food's ability to elevate blood glucose levels is referred to as its glycemic index. Simple sugars have a high glycemic index because they cause a very rapid increase in blood glucose levels. Larger, more complex carbohydrates, such as starches, have a low glycemic index because they cause a gradual increase in blood glucose levels.

High glycemic index foods—foods that contain a lot of sugar—will tend to increase your storage of body fat. The reason for this is that each fat cell in your body can respond to insulin, take glucose out of the blood, and store it; but instead of storing the extra glucose as glycogen like the muscles and liver do, these cells store the excess glucose as fat. The higher your blood glucose rises, the more glucose will be stored in your fat cells. To minimize the amount of carbohydrate that ends up being stored as fat, it is important that you consume low glycemic index foods such as whole grains, pastas, nuts, seeds, tomatoes, beans, grapefruit, apples, and peas.

Proteins

Proteins are required to maintain the normal structure and function of the body. Whereas carbohydrates, especially glucose, are the primary fuel source for the body, proteins are used as the primary building blocks of the body tissues like muscle, bone, and connective tissue. In addition, enzymes, antibodies, hemoglobin, and even your DNA are all made from protein.

Proteins are made up of twenty different amino acids. Twelve of these amino acids can be synthesized in your body and therefore do not need to come from your diet. These are called the non-essential amino acids. The other eight amino acids are essential amino acids and need to come from your diet, including isoleucine, leucine, lysine, methionine, phenyl-alanine, threonine, tryptophan and valine. If you do not get enough of these amino acids in your diet, your body cannot repair itself: your immune system can't do its job properly, your metabolism decreases, and you feel sluggish, depressed, and tired. The primary sources of these amino acids are from protein sources such as meat, fish, cheese, eggs, soy, dairy products, beans, and legumes.

Before your body can use the protein in your food, it must first break down the protein to its individual amino acids. Digestion of protein begins in the stomach where acids and proteolytic enzymes begin the process of releasing amino acids from the protein. Some amino acids are absorbed directly through the stomach lining and enter into the blood stream. The remaining protein then enters the small intestine where digestion is completed.

Once the amino acids enter the blood, the body can use them to build red blood cells, muscle tissue, immune factors, or whatever else the body needs. But there's a catch! All twenty amino acids must be present in the blood in the proper ratios in order for the body to manufacture new proteins—to repair muscles, for example. If one amino acid is missing or is present in a very limited quantity, then that amino acid becomes the limiting factor to protein synthesis. For this reason, it is best to eat proteins that have all of the amino acids that the body needs.

The proteins in some foods have amino acid profiles that very closely match the ratios that the human body needs, such as eggs, dairy, and meat. These proteins are said to have a high biological value (BV). Eggs are considered to have the highest biological value and are used as the standard to which all other proteins are compared. In the Biological Value of Protein chart, you will see that eggs have a BV score of 100. The 100 signifies that approximately 100 percent of the protein in eggs can be metabolized by the body because it so closely matches the amino acid profile of the human body.

Other foods eaten by themselves, such as grains, vegetables, and beans, have amino acid profiles that do not match the body's needs as well. These are lower biological quality proteins and have lower BV scores. However, if you paired together lentils and rice, all amino acids would be present to make a complete protein. Other complete amino acid combinations include legumes or vegetables and grains; legumes or vegetables and nuts; and mushrooms and vegetables.

You will notice that whey (milk) protein concentrate has a BV of 104. Is it possible to have a 104 percent of the milk proteins absorbed? Well, no. When the standard of biological value was initially set, egg protein had the best amino acid profile of any protein known at the time, so eggs were made the standard and given a value of 100. Since then, it was discovered that highly concentrated whey protein from milk actually had a slightly better amino acid profile than eggs. Instead of changing the standard to whey, it was decided to just give whey protein a score of more than 100.

The other measure of the overall quality of protein is how much of the protein can be digested by your body: this is its Percentage of Digestion (PD) score. Some proteins such as bone, cartilage, and tendon may have a high biological value because of their amino acid profiles, but are completely non-digestible—therefore your body cannot absorb the amino acids they contain. When you are cutting back on your overall food intake in an effort to lose weight, it is important to eat higher biological value proteins, as well as those with the highest digestibility (PD).

Biological Value of Protein Chart

Source	Protein (g)	Biological Value
Chicken breast (2.8 oz, 79 g)	26	79
Tuna (3.0 oz, 85 g)	24	83
Egg (1 whole)	6	100
Milk (1%, 1 cup)	8	91
Lean beef (2.5 oz, 72 g)	22	80
Lentils (1 cup)	16	50
Red kidney beans (1 cup)	15	50
Bread (1 slice, 25 g)	2	54
Rice (1 cup)	4	59
Pasta (1 cup)	4	54
Oatmeal (1 cup)	13	55
Whey concentrate	--	104

Proteins have an added advantage over carbohydrates in that they don't cause a rapid increase in blood glucose levels: they are low glycemic index foods. Proteins will increase your body's metabolism more than carbohydrates and fats; they also provide the building blocks for many mood-elevating neurotransmitters, such as phenylalanine and tryptophan.

Proteins are critical for building lean muscle tissue and for maintaining stable blood glucose levels, immune function, and normal brain chemistry. Since proteins with a higher biological value more closely match the needs of the body, eating higher biological value proteins has the advantage of giving you the greatest amount of usable protein for the number of calories consumed.

Fats

Of the three major components of food, fats are certainly the most misunderstood and the most vilified. Fat is not the bad thing that it is often made out to be. Dietary fats are necessary for the proper absorption of fat-soluble vitamins, and scientists recently discovered that some fats in the diet are used for sending signals to the brain to control how much you eat. In fact, all of the cells in your body are surrounded by a membrane of fat. That's why you can go swimming and not dissolve in the water. Your brain, spinal cord, and entire nervous system are largely made from fat, as well as many of your hormones, such as testosterone and estrogen. Fat provides your body with a store of energy and insulation from the cold, and it protects your organs from physical damage. In fact, next to water, fat is the most abundant substance in the human body, ideally averaging about 10 to 20 percent of a person's total body weight.

Dietary fats come in several forms: saturated fats, polyunsaturated fats, monounsaturated fats, and cholesterol. Saturated fats are the fats that most Americans think they need to avoid to protect their hearts from disease. In major prospective studies to date, however, there is little relation between saturated fat intake and the risk of coronary heart disease. In fact, studies have shown that the fat in clogged arteries is only about 26 percent saturated: the rest is unsaturated. Saturated fats actually play a crucial role in building and maintaining healthy bones. In order for the skeletal structure to absorb calcium, saturated fat must make up a significant amount of daily dietary fat. In addition, saturated fats made up of short and medium-chain fatty acids, such as coconut oil, have antimicrobial properties, meaning they help protect your digestive tract against dangerous micro-organisms.

It is generally recommended that daily intake of fat not exceed 30 percent of total calories consumed, and that saturated fat should make up 20 to 30 percent of total fat. Choose lower-fat meats like chicken and turkey over processed meats with high levels of saturated fats, and use only moderate amounts of dairy products (like cheese, whole milk, cream, and butter).

The most frequently consumed polyunsaturated fats are vegetable oils derived from soy, corn, and safflower. Certain polyunsaturated fats, such as the omega-3 fatty acids, help to decrease serum cholesterol, both LDL and HDL, and will help to decrease inflammation in the body. These good fats can be found in high quantities in flax oil, walnuts, fish, and algae. It is very important that polyunsaturated oils that have been turned into trans-fats during the process of hydrogenation be avoided all together.

Polyunsaturated fats tend to be liquid at room temperature, whereas saturated fats are usually solid. In order to have polyunsaturated fats last longer without turning rancid, food manufacturers devised the hydrogenation process that solidifies these fats. These new trans-fats have been linked to cancer, atherosclerosis, diabetes, obesity, immune system dysfunction, low-birth-weight babies, birth defects, decreased visual acuity, sterility, difficulty in lactation, and problems with bones and tendons. You will find hydrogenated oils in the ingredient list on packaged foods such as cookies, crackers, candy, chips, baked goods, and margarine.

Monounsaturated fats, on the other hand, not only decrease your bad LDL cholesterol, but they also help raise your good HDL cholesterol! Using olives, olive oil, canola oil, peanut oil, avocados, and nuts in the preparation of your daily meals is the simplest way to introduce monounsaturates into your diet.

Cholesterol is a waxy fat that is found exclusively in animal foods—beef, chicken, fish, turkey, eggs, and dairy. Years ago it was believed that consuming cholesterol in your diet led to an increase in your blood cholesterol, but this turned out to not be the case. Dietary cholesterol has very little, if any, impact on the blood cholesterol level of most people. The major contributors to "high cholesterol" are eating too much saturated fat, being overweight, and not getting enough exercise.

Calories

A calorie is a measure of the energy content of food. Calories are what your body uses to keep your heart pumping, keep your lungs breathing, allow your mind to think, and give your muscles the energy needed to move you around. Carbohydrates and protein each provide four calories per gram, fats provide nine calories per gram, and alcohol provides approximately seven calories per gram. In other words, ounce for ounce, proteins and carbohydrates give you fewer than half of the calories of fat. The high caloric value of fat is why high-fat foods, such as cream cheese and fried foods, are so high in calories. It is important to remember that calories are not your enemy. As strange as it may seem, if you don't eat enough food, it will be harder for you to lose weight. This is because too much calorie restriction slows down your metabolism.

Maintaining a healthy body composition is a balancing act between the calories you consume and the calories you burn. We have spent some time discussing the main sources of energy in your diet—carbohydrates, proteins, and fats. Let's take a quick look at the other side of the equation: how your body burns the calories you consume.

Your body burns calories in two ways: your basal energy expenditure (also known as your basal metabolic rate) and your activity level. The biggest user of calories is your basal energy expenditure (BEE), which is the energy used by your organs to keep your body alive and to build muscles, bone, and connective tissue. Your BEE is responsible for burning up to three-fourths of all the calories you burn in one day.

Activity is the other way in which you burn calories. Depending on how active you are, activity can make up as little as fifteen percent, or as much as thirty-five percent of the total calories you burn in a day.

Three Things Everyone Should Do

Drink More Water and Cleanse the System

Water is the single most abundant nutrient in the body, accounting for around 60 to 65 percent of your total weight. It is also the least forgiving of all the nutrients you consume. You can survive for weeks without food, but for only a couple of days without water. Water is responsible for the transport of nutrients, oxygen, and waste products, as well as for regulating your body temperature and serving as the medium in which all of your body's chemical reactions take place. Most people do not drink enough pure clean water.

Drinking an adequate amount of clean water every day is one of the most overlooked but simplest ways of keeping your body healthy. Water is used to help the body cleanse itself from toxins and metabolic waste. Although drinking water has become more popular over the past several years, many people still do not consume enough water. Instead, they drink coffee, tea, juices, and soft drinks and figure that they get enough fluids.

It is true that when you drink these beverages you are consuming water. However, along with the water, you are also consuming a lot of other stuff that the body will need to ultimately eliminate, so the potential benefit of the water is somewhat negated. To make matters worse, drinks that contain caffeine, such as coffee, tea, and soft drinks, actually cause more water loss than the amount of water they contain, resulting in a net loss of water.

Ideally, the average person should consume around ten cups of water per day, or just over a half gallon. Some of this water is found in the food and beverages you consume, so you don't have to drink an entire half-gallon of water every day. I recommend you buy a 1.5 liter bottle of water from the local grocery store and to drink at least that amount of water every day. If you exercise heavily, you will have to drink more. By drinking enough water, you will be helping your body to remain healthy. It is by far the cheapest health insurance you can buy.

Another way to flush the system of toxins is to periodically cleanse the body with special detoxifying diets. Our cells trap waste and destructive substances that come from consuming sugar, refined white flour carbohydrates, trans-fats, alcohol, and caffeine. To give the liver and your other organs a chance to eliminate these toxins, you may choose to eat only nutrient-dense fruits and vegetables on certain days. Other methods of elimination include probiotics (good bacteria such as lactobacillus and bifidobacteria), useful for renewing your intestinal health.

Eat More Fruits and Vegetables

People know that they should get more fruit and vegetables in their diet, but most people don't do it. It seems lately that the four major food groups of the American diet have gone from dairy, vegetables, grains, and meat to sugar, fat, salt, and caffeine. Because of the easy availability of fast foods and snack foods, we have lost our taste for fruits and vegetables, especially vegetables. It is not uncommon for many people to go for weeks without consuming a single serving of fresh vegetables. This is no way to achieve health.

The human body evolved with a diet high in fruits and vegetables, and it is dependent on many of the compounds unique to plant foods in order to operate correctly. If you don't consume enough of these plant compounds, your energy level will suffer along with your overall health.

By eating more fruits and vegetables, you will also increase your fiber intake. Fiber is necessary for bowel regulation and for weight-loss. Fiber is filling without being fattening: it requires more chewing, and the prolonged chewing, besides pre-digesting the food, satisfies the appetite. It will slow down the absorption of fat from what you eat, creating another weight-control benefit.

Fiber also acts like a biological broom, sweeping potentially toxic waste products through the intestines more quickly. Most people are shocked at how much better they feel when they cut down on the fast foods and snack foods and increase their fruit and vegetable intake.

If you find it difficult to fit several servings of fruits and vegetables into your routine every day, although it is not as good as actually eating real fruits and vegetables, you may find it helpful to supplement your diet with what is called a greens-supplement: this is a highly concentrated powder of fruits, vegetables, and antioxidants. Ultimately, increasing your consumption of fruits and vegetables is the best way to improve your overall health. The key is to make it part of your lifestyle—to make it a new habit.

Take a Supplement

A nutrition professor once posed a challenge to his class: construct a 2,000 calorie-per-day diet that met the Recommended Dietary Allowances (RDA) for vitamins and minerals without the use of supplements. After all, we have always heard that if you eat a well-balanced diet, you don't need to take vitamin supplements, right? Well, this professor was putting that statement to the test.

To everyone's surprise, not one student was able to come up with a sustainable daily diet that met the minimum requirements for mineral intake. Getting the minimum vitamin intake was relatively easy. The challenge was getting enough of a few very important minerals, especially zinc. Unless you eat oysters or dark turkey meat every day, it is impossible to get the minimum RDA of zinc through diet alone.

So, it is not possible to get everything that you need from the food we eat. But how could this be? Certainly people have lived on this planet for a long time and must have been able to get everything they needed from their diet. The answer has to do with modern farming techniques, fertilizers, and environmental stresses.

Following the Second World War, chemical manufacturers were sitting on huge stockpiles of phosphates and nitrates that were initially intended for use in explosives. They discovered that when they spread these same phosphates and nitrates on the soil where plants were growing, the plants grew bigger and looked healthier. Thus began the boom of the fertilizer industry.

The problem with modern fertilizers is that they don't replace soil trace minerals, such as chromium, zinc, and copper, as do cow manure and other natural fertilizers. Over time, these trace minerals become more and more depleted from the soil and, consequently, our food supply becomes more depleted as well. The bottom line is that in order to get enough trace minerals in our diet to at least meet the minimum RDAs, it is necessary to take a good quality supplement.

Another good reason for taking a multivitamin is the substantial evidence that taking doses of a class of nutrients called antioxidants (especially vitamins A, C, E, and selenium) far exceeding the RDA minimums can help prevent heart disease, help to mitigate some of the detrimental effects of environmental pollutants, and help promote healthy immune function.

Essential fatty acids are another example of a supplement that is necessary to take on a consistent basis because these are difficult to consume in our daily diets. Look for quality supplements from professional grade manufacturers. Often people become confused at which supplements to purchase because most consumers don't know how to tell the difference between them. They figure if it has the name on the label than that's the supplement to buy. Experts will tell you that all supplements are not the same. Ask your wellness doctor what brand of supplements they recommend.

Making Sense of It All

The foods you eat on a daily basis have a tremendous impact on your overall health. If you eat all-natural, health-giving foods, your body will be healthier. If you eat junk, your physical health will suffer. Remember that your body's only source for its building materials is the food that goes into your mouth.

In addition to eating a wide variety of natural, health-giving foods, you may also benefit from taking a good quality vitamin supplement and drinking plenty of water. The vitamin supplement ensures that all of the metabolic processes in your body can be performed effectively and the water helps to keep the metabolic waste and toxins flushed out of your system.

In summary, the most important concepts about nutrition to remember are:

1. *Make sure you have a healthy relationship with food. That doesn't mean that you should have a love affair with food. It means that you should eat for nourishment and enjoy the pleasure of good food. Too often, people eat out of habit or guilt or for other emotional reasons related to a low self-esteem.*

2. *One of the simplest concepts to remember about healthy eating habits is to think of healthy eating in the opposite way that you would your financial budget. Do your best to make sure that you exercise and burn more calories than you consume every day; that way your body doesn't get into the habit of saving calories. You have a lot more flexibility in what you eat when your body is in the habit of burning calories on a consistent basis.*

12

Healthy Thinking

Anna O. was Dr. Joseph Breuer's patient from 1880 through 1882. She was twenty-one years old and spent most of her time nursing her ailing father. She developed a bad cough that proved to have no physical basis and soon after, began to develop some speech difficulties; eventually she became mute. After her father died, she developed an unusual set of problems. She lost the feeling in her hands and feet, developed some paralysis, and began to have involuntary spasms. She also had visual hallucinations and tunnel vision. But when specialists were consulted, no physical causes for these problems could be found.

This was one of the case studies from Sigmund Freud's *Aetiology of Hysteria* published in 1896. The case study goes on to tell about how Anna O. was eventually cured of her physical maladies, not by medicine, but through treating her thoughts and emotions. This was one of the first documented cases describing the connection between our thoughts and emotions and our physical health.

It has now been over a hundred years since the discovery of the mind-body link, and Western medicine still does not really pay much attention to the place of thoughts and emotions in human health. In a health care system that focuses on drugs and quick fixes, thoughts and emotions are seen as too ambiguous and too variable to be important. In fact, the use of pharmaceutical drugs such as antidepressants to treat emotional problems really indicates that modern medicine has put the cart before the horse. They assume that we feel a certain way BECAUSE of our physical condition, rather than understand that how we feel is THE CAUSE of our physical condition.

There was an interesting study conducted at UCLA in the early 1990s where 14 professional actors were recruited to study the effects of emotion on the immune system. During the study, the actors were told which mood state they would be experiencing. They then read the appropriate scenario, which was about 100 words long, and were told to create and experience a realistic mood by developing the scene and verbally and behaviorally acting it out while seated. Actors were encouraged to use their own personal memories to intensify the experience.

Once the actors were in a particular emotional state, the researchers drew blood to measure any physical changes that may be associated with particular emotional states. What they found surprised everyone. Simply by shifting from one emotional state to another, the actors could stimulate or suppress their immune function. Subsequent studies have measured all kinds of physical changes that result from emotional states, such as changes in hormone levels, brain chemistry, blood sugar levels, and even the ability to heal properly.

In fact, the mind-body connection is so strong that an entire field of science has emerged called psychoneuroimmunology. More and more scientific studies are published proving the idea that thoughts and emotions have a powerful influence over our physical health. This is one of the reasons why people are much more likely to get sick during job changes, holidays, and other stressful times, or why people who are depressed have a much higher risk of developing cancer.

How can emotions affect our immunity or resistance to disease? Research shows that the brain can release hormones and other chemicals that affect white blood cells and other parts of the immune system. Though the chemicals also have other functions, they are a link between our thoughts and our ability to resist diseases.

For example, when people react to stresses with fear, their brains send a "danger" message to the body. Hormones are released to raise blood pressure and prepare muscles for quick action, as if to fight or flee from danger. The stress hormones also depress the disease-resistance system, and over time, can damage the brain, heart, and digestive tract.

Thoughts can cause physical abnormalities such as ulcers, indigestion, nervousness, and high blood pressure. Thoughts can also depress the immune system, which leads to a wide variety of diseases. Whether a person experiences poor health, and how soon, depends on that person's heredity, environment, diet, and behavior.

An Australian study in the late 1970s showed that when one spouse dies, the other experiences a weakened immune system. This helps explain why grieving spouses have more diseases and a higher death rate than others of similar age.

Other studies have shown that heart patients who are depressed have more heart problems than happier heart patients; in these cases, depression was a better predictor of problems than physical measurements were.

Cancer is more common in people who suffer a major emotional loss, repress anger, and feel helpless. Cancer patients who express their emotions rather than denying them seem to recover more quickly. The link between emotion and cancer is so strong that some psychological tests are better predictors of cancer than physical exams are.

This does not mean that everyone who has cancer or some other disease has simply thought it upon himself. There are many factors involved in disease; even the best attitude is not going to prevent ill effects from genetic malfunctions and some chemical and biological hazards.

A new study shows physical proof of how one emotional factor—a strong and happy marriage—can be a boon to your health. According to the study, physical wounds take much longer to heal in marriages marred by hostility and conflict than those in which couples build a more pleasurable home life.

Get Positive!

Just as negative emotions can weaken the body's resistance, positive emotions can strengthen it, or at least allow it to function normally. The simple act of deciding to be happier and focus on the positive will improve your health. In fact, this phenomenon of your thoughts affecting your physical health is so strong that all medical studies have to be designed with it in mind. Researchers call this phenomenon "the placebo effect."

Many people believe that the term "placebo effect" means that the effect is only imagined—that it is not real. But this couldn't be further from the truth. Medical studies have to include a control group—people who receive placebos instead of the medicine being studied—because the simple act of people making the decision to take action to improve their health leads to measurable physical improvement in their condition. To determine how much of an effect a particular medicine had, the researchers have to take the measured change in the group who underwent the particular therapy and subtract out the amount of change seen in the placebo group. Otherwise, there is no way to know whether a particular treatment was beneficial or whether it was merely the change in attitude in the study subjects that made the difference. In many instances, the placebo effect turns out to be stronger than the treatment itself!

The point is that if you want to have a healthy body, you need to have healthy thoughts and emotions. Just as it is important to avoid toxic chemicals, it is also necessary to avoid toxic thoughts to enjoy optimal health.

Relaxation

Today, we are more stressed-out than ever before. The stress of careers, deadlines, conflicts, and demands on our time and money take a huge toll on our health and well-being. Just as a chain tends to break at its weakest link, we exhibit stress and strain in the weakest areas of our bodies.

Stress basically comes in three forms of overload. We encounter physical stress, emotional stress, and chemical stress. In fact, we are subject to all three almost all the time. When we overload, it always manifests in symptoms at our weakest link. Some of us develop ulcers, others migraines, others low back pain, others insomnia, and so forth.

It may not be possible to remove all of the stress from life. There are, however, safe, all-natural, and effective stress reduction strategies that help offset the bad effects that stress produces and strengthen the function of the nervous and immune systems at the same time, so you can make stress your friend, not your enemy.

After decades of research, it is clear that the negative effects associated with stress are real. Although you may not always be able to avoid stressful situations, there are a number of things that you can do to reduce the effect that stress has on your body. The first is relaxation. Learning to relax doesn't have to be difficult. Here are some simple techniques to help get you started on your way to tranquility.

Positive Affirmations

We function a lot like computers: garbage in produces garbage out, while great stuff in produces great stuff out. We talk to ourselves far more than we talk to others. In fact, most experts agree that about eighty percent of all conversations we have are with ourselves. All too often, we talk to ourselves with anger, fear, belittlement, and negativity. "I knew there wouldn't be any parking," or, "I knew that they were going to be mad at me," or, "I am always depressed this time of year," or even, "I just can't seem to do anything right"—these are examples of the kind of inner-talk we play over and over again in our minds. We acknowledge our ability to manifest our inner-thinking and yet the majority of our inner-thinking is negative and demeaning.

This raises a very important question. If we are powerful enough to manifest our negative thoughts, why can't we also manifest our positive thoughts? The answer is that we can. In order to create positive thoughts instead of negative ones, we must decide in advance to be proactive and to discipline ourselves to take out the old mental program of negativity and immediately replace it with the new mental program of being positive and kind. I have found the best way to do this is through the use of affirmations.

Affirmations are positive self-talk designed to help you create the life of your dreams. Using affirmations on a daily basis is one of the simplest and easiest action steps you can take to get what you want out of life and to reduce stress, fear, and depression. Making positive, affirming statements to yourself will change your self-image, raise your self-esteem, and create an attitude of expectancy.

Here are some of the keys that allow you to maximize the power of your daily affirmations:

- *Affirmations should be written down. This allows you to crystallize your thoughts and gives you a reference to refer back to daily.*

- *Affirmations should be in the first person and in the current time frame. They should always contain the word "I" and be in the "now" time frame, as they are the truth, told in advance. Remember the rule, "To Become, Act As If."*

- *Affirmations are best done in the morning to start your day or in the evening before going to sleep. This helps to program your subconscious mind with positive thoughts.*

- *Affirmations, either memorized or read, need to be said aloud with emotion. This is necessary to open the trap door between your educated and innate mind.*

Let me share some possible affirmations with you to get you thinking properly about creating your own. Remember that you can and should create affirmations for all parts of your life. Affirm professionally, spiritually, financially, and in all other areas. For example:

"Today is a great day and I have the opportunity to show up as the best me ever! I am an irresistible magnet with the absolute power to attract into my life everything that I desire. My life is a huge success!

I am committed to constant and never ending personal improvement, and I take massive action steps to create the future as I want it. I will do whatever it takes to become the winner I know I can be.

My beliefs create my reality! I choose robust health, abundant wealth, constant happiness and eternal love. I attract, heal, and positively influence the lives of people in my community. I think big thoughts, relish small pleasures, and handle all setbacks gracefully.

I give thanks for the opportunity to serve humanity, and I willingly accept the rewards being sent to me by an abundant universe. I am deeply grateful for all I create and receive. My life is now in total balance and … I am a master!"

To print a copy of this affirmation, go to

DiscoverWellnessCenter.com

Relaxed Breathing

Have you ever noticed how you breathe when you're stressed? Stress typically causes rapid, shallow breathing. This kind of breathing sustains other aspects of the stress response, such as rapid heart rate and perspiration. If you can get control of your breathing, the spiraling effects of acute stress will automatically become less intense. Relaxed breathing, also called diaphragmatic breathing, can help you.

Practice this basic technique twice daily and whenever you feel tense. Follow these steps:

- *Inhale. With your mouth closed and your shoulders relaxed, inhale as slowly and deeply as you can to the count of six. As you do that, push your stomach out. Allow the air to fill your diaphragm.*

- *Hold. Keep the air in your lungs as you slowly count to four.*

- *Exhale. Release the air through your mouth as you slowly count to six.*

- *Repeat. Complete the inhale-hold-exhale cycle three to five times.*

Progressive Muscle Relaxation

The goal of progressive muscle relaxation is to reduce the tension in your muscles. First, find a quiet place where you'll be free from interruption. Loosen tight clothing and remove your glasses or contacts if you'd like.

Tense each muscle group for at least five seconds and then relax for at least 30 seconds. Repeat before moving to the next muscle group.

- *Face. Squint your eyes tightly, wrinkle your nose and mouth, clench your teeth, and pull back the corners of your mouth toward your ears, feeling the tension in the center of your face. Relax. Repeat.*

- *Neck. Gently touch your chin to your chest. Feel the pull in the back of your neck as it spreads into your head. Relax. Repeat.*

- *Shoulders. Pull your shoulders up toward your ears, feeling the tension in your shoulders, head, neck, and upper back. Relax. Repeat.*

- *Upper arms. Pull your arms back and press your elbows in toward the sides of your body. Try not to tense your lower arms. Feel the tension in your arms, shoulders, and into your back. Relax. Repeat.*

- *Hands and forearms. Make a tight fist and pull up your wrists. Feel the tension in your hands, knuckles, and lower arms. Relax. Repeat.*

- *Chest, shoulders, and upper back. Pull your shoulders back as if you're trying to make your shoulder blades touch. Relax. Repeat.*

- *Stomach. Pull your stomach in toward your spine, tightening your abdominal muscles. Relax. Repeat.*

- *Upper legs. Squeeze your knees together and lift your legs up off the chair or from wherever you're relaxing. Feel the tension in your thighs. Relax. Repeat.*

- *Lower legs. Raise your feet toward the ceiling while flexing them toward your body. Feel the tension in your calves. Relax. Repeat.*

- *Feet. Turn your feet inward and curl your toes up and out. Relax. Repeat.*

Perform progressive muscle relaxation at least once or twice each day to get the maximum benefit. Each session should last about ten minutes.

Autogenic Relaxation

"Autogenic" means something that comes from within you. During this type of relaxation, you repeat words or suggestions in your mind to help you relax and reduce the tension in your muscles. Find a peaceful place where you'll be free of interruptions. Then follow these steps:

- *Choose a focus word, phrase, or image you find relaxing. This is called a mantra.*

- *Sit quietly in a comfortable position and close your eyes.*

- *Breathe slowly and naturally, focusing on your mantra.*

- *Continue for 10-20 minutes. If your mind wanders, that's okay. Gently return your focus to your breathing and the word, phrase, or image you selected.*

Listen to Soothing Sounds

If you have about ten minutes and a quiet room, you can take a mental vacation almost anytime. Consider these two types of relaxation CDs or tapes to help you unwind, rest your mind or take a visual journey to a peaceful place.

• *Spoken word. These CDs use spoken suggestions to guide your meditation, educate you on stress reduction, or take you on an imaginary visual journey to a peaceful place.*

• *Soothing music or nature sounds. Music has the power to affect your thoughts and feelings. Soft, soothing music can help you relax and lower your stress level.*

No one CD works for everyone, so try several CDs to find which works best for you. When possible, listen to samples in the store. Consider asking your friends or a trusted professional for recommendations.

Relationships with Others

Relationships are important for good emotional health. Numerous studies have shown that people who have close friends and intimate relationships suffer less pain, are healthier and happier, and live longer. In fact, the simple act of petting a dog, holding a child, or seeing someone you love causes a decrease in stress hormones in the blood, decreases blood pressure, and calms the mind. So, if you want to be healthy, stay connected to others.

As the author Dr. Tedd Koren says, "Emotional health is also dependent on being connected—to yourself and others. The more connected you are to yourself the more you can connect with others and the more fulfilling your connections (relationships). The more relationships in your life the more happiness, joy, hope, optimism, and vitality you will have; the healthier and longer you will live and the quicker you will recover from physical and emotional traumas and illness."

Relationship with Your Self

Your relationship with your self is the most important relationship because, as they say, wherever you go, there you are. Wellness begins with "being" well first and then "doing" things to be well. If you do not address who you are "being," then just "doing" things will not make you well. A simple way to remember this is that we refer to ourselves as human beings, not human doings.

Dr. Sue Morter, a wellness expert and one of the developers of Morter Health Systems teaches about self-esteem and healthy thinking in an extremely effective and practical manner. She explains how the body is the caboose of our self. It is who we are, how we think, and the story we tell about our life that impacts our physical health and well-being. Her inspirational high-energy seminars begin by asking the simple question "Are you living well?" "Yes, I AM" the audience proclaims in an effort to understand that living well begins with making the self-declaration that "I choose to be well." Her powerful message is communicated beautifully through simple stories that explain insightful metaphors for attaining things that are important for us to have in our lives. For example, if you were going to a party that you knew would not have the food or drink you wanted, what would you do, she asks? Just "bring it" the audience responds. That is what you do, too, to begin the process of "being" well: you bring it forward in your awareness.

If the idea that our thinking affects our health seems far-fetched, there is a really simple way to illustrate how this is true. If I were to ask you to open your hand and then close it into a fist and you could do this, you would be illustrating exactly the same concept of how your mind or your thinking causes your body to move and to function. Perhaps you may think that is too simple.

What if I were to show up on your door step and tell you that you had just won the *Discover Wellness, How Staying Healthy Can Make You Rich* sweepstakes grand prize of $100 million: do you think your breathing would change? Might your heart rate change at least a little bit? How about your blood pressure? That's because your awareness or consciousness affects your physical body, and it works both for you and against you.

Most people don't realize this cause-and-effect relationship and therefore reverse it by determining what they should think based on how they feel. "I AM so sick and tired of all this," people exclaim. "I AM in pain," "I AM angry," and so on. It is completely up to us to determine who we choose to be and what we choose to feel, and those choices are at the root of how our body responds.

Based on this understanding of how health and wellness come from within, who else can we expect to manifest it for us in our lives? It is our personal responsibility to become self-aware, or as Dr. Sue Morter once again so simply puts it, "We must be present to win." We must live in the present in a state of gratitude and appreciation for our lives and circumstances in it. Our relationship with our self is our self-responsibility and the basis of intentional living and manifesting our innate wellness.

SPECIAL SECTION

Perspectives on Wellness

By Dr. Dennis Perman, D.C.
Vice President
The Masters Circle

What's the main difference between standard medical care and wellness care? Standard medical care seeks to treat a symptom by adding something from the outside —a medication, a surgery, or procedure. Wellness care, on the other hand, seeks to turn on the natural healing ability, not by adding something to the system, but by removing anything that might interfere with normal function, trusting that the body would know what to do if nothing were interfering with it.

Inside Out vs. Outside In

If a patient has high blood pressure, a standard medical approach would be to choose a drug that lowers blood pressure and ask the patient to take the drug. This may serve to lower the blood pressure, but it ignores the underlying cause that is making the blood pressure high and runs the risk of side effects complicating the person's recovery. Whether the cause is a nutritional issue, faulty control by the nervous system, or a manifestation of stress, the medication decreases the blood pressure, leaving the problem causing the symptom of high blood pressure unaddressed.

The Wellness Approach

Wellness is a state of optimal conditions for normal function ... and then some. The wellness approach looks for underlying causes of any disturbance or disruption (which may or may not be causing symptoms at the time) and make whatever interventions and lifestyle adjustments that would optimize the conditions for normal function. That environment encourages natural healing, and minimizes the need for invasive treatment, which should be administered only when absolutely necessary. When the body is working properly, it tends to heal effectively, no matter what the condition. When the body heals well and maintains itself well, then there is another level of health that goes beyond "asymp-tomatic" or "pain-free," which reveals an open-ended opportunity for vitality, vibrant health, and an enhanced experience of life.

This is true for mental and emotional health as well as physical health. While some people may suffer psychological disorders, creating an atmosphere of mental and emotional wellness will address all but the most serious problems.

What is Wellness Psychology?

Wellness psychology is the study of mental and emotional wellness—in other words, the way to create conditions of thinking and feeling that are consistent with healthy living. Wellness psychology is a way of responding to the challenges of life with positive expectancy and self-esteem, based on the awareness that our natural state is harmony and inner peace, if we can reduce or eliminate whatever is interfering with that state.

Wellness psychology is based more on lifestyle decisions than on the treatment by a professional. Learning to interpret the events of your life with positive realism gives you a perspective from which you can assign uplifting meanings to those events. Tony Robbins says, "Nothing has any meaning but the meaning you give it;" and putting a positive spin on things sets an internal environment that is more likely to encourage overall wellness.

But there's more to wellness psychology than just positive thinking. Rather than waiting around for mental and emotional symptoms, you can be proactive and develop habits that make you mentally and emotionally healthier on an ongoing basis.

Wellness Choices and Decisions

Scientists tell us that much of our self-talk is negative, so learning to be kind and supportive in your mental chatter is a direct step toward a well mind. Practice saying constructive things to yourself, like "I'm a good person," "today's going to be a great day," "I can do this;" simple stuff like that. One of the most powerful tools you can use is saying affirmations, positive statements spoken aloud daily that focus your mind and establish a consistent tone of empowerment.

Visualizing or imagining a desirable future helps to promote wellness by creating feelings of excitement, fun, and positive expectancy. It also sensitizes us to anything we come across in real life that reminds us of our vision, so we start to pick up on distinctions we might otherwise miss. There is even considerable evidence to suggest that visualization influences what happens; but one way or another, using your imagination is a constructive habit that adds to the wellness experience.

Setting goals can be very helpful, to focus the mind on productive activities and enhance self-esteem and personal growth. Success is a frequent by-product of a well mind, since the energy used to deal with mental and emotional issues can be reclaimed and reinvested in more fulfilling outcomes and achievements.

Meditation and prayer are useful wellness habits, too. Getting quiet inside and connecting with your higher self or more formally giving thanks and appreciation to your Maker for your many blessings are tried and true ways for adding to the wellness equation.

Watching your nutrition also contributes to mental and emotional wellness. Sugar and caffeine may make you edgy, and dehydration can cause psychological unrest, so drinking sufficient water is a crucial wellness habit. Vitamins and minerals play a major role in mind function, so a well-balanced nutritional regime, with lots of high water-content foods like fresh fruits and vegetables, aids your body chemistry and enhances your psychological condition. Also, avoid foods with high concentrations of hormones, antibiotics, or additives, which may irritate your nervous system and cause symptoms.

Physical activity is essential for a wellness lifestyle, and it has a profound positive impact on your perception of reality. Breathing, stretching, or walking can both stimulate and relax you, and more vigorous activity like aerobics, running, or weight training keeps your machinery operating at peak efficiency. Programs like *Body-For-Life* by Bill Phillips that incorporate exercise, proper diet, and an optimistic outlook are likely to promote wellness between your ears as well as around your midsection.

Alignment is the missing link of wellness psychology. Alignment of physical structures like the spine and nervous system work hand in hand with alignment of the thinking, values, and beliefs, to formulate the best possible internal environment, leading to optimum function and physiological freedom.

Identity

The major distinction of wellness psychology is that it is largely a manifestation of your identity, who you believe yourself to be. If you consider yourself a well person, that goes a long way toward producing well habits and a well mind. Your identity is your self-image, your self-concept, your beliefs, and your values. Choosing beliefs and values that are consistent with well behaviors leads to a well mind.

For example, if you were told as a child that if you washed your hair and went outside with a wet head, you'd get sick, there's a good chance you either don't do that, or when you do, you either get sick or worry that you will. This belief, imposed on you by well-meaning but misguided advisors, has no grounding in fact; so merely noticing when you dredge up stuff like this, and challenging it to see if it's really true for you can eliminate interference with normal function caused by faulty thinking. You'll actually heal better and faster when you catch yourself in these limiting beliefs and adjust them.

Your identity is based on your sense of self, which largely came from the beliefs of such well-intentioned people who shaped your early life — as Dr. Larry Markson says, your Mothers, Fathers, Teachers, and Preachers: MFTP. Discovering the beliefs that prevent you from expressing yourself as you wish and replacing them with beliefs that empower you and help you grow lead to a well psychology.

Examine your values, what you consider to be important, and be sure they match your ideals. Honoring your innermost needs and wants instead of denying them creates an internal environment of self-acceptance, integrity, and inner peace. Love, respect, honesty, freedom—everyone has a different formula, and investigating yours can help you feel more comfortable in your own skin.

Personality

The technical end of wellness psychology encourages normal responses to the challenges of life, rather than treating mental and emotional conditions. Understanding the concept of personality makes this approach clearer.

People tend to have patterns of behavior, some of which work better than others, but the patterns usually persist until they are broken or replaced. Noticing these patterns and evaluating them to see if they are constructive or destructive, then shifting the patterns accordingly, makes wellness more accessible.

There are many ways to group or evaluate personality type. People tend to favor one of the three major ways the brain processes—visual (seeing), auditory (hearing), and kinesthetic (feeling)—and each group has common patterns of behavior. Or you can divide people by personality style, into drivers, expressives, analyticals, and amiables. You can notice typical behaviors, known as metaprograms, such as moving toward benefits versus moving away from consequences or having an internal versus external frame of reference. There are more technical systems of personality, like Myers-Briggs or the enneagram, which offer deeper understanding and pathways for personal growth.

Why is personality important? Healthy people express themselves consistent with their personality types, and those types vary greatly, so there is a wide spectrum of normal behaviors that could be considered well behaviors. Knowing yourself and understanding others with whom you have a relationship can give you insight into the unique nature of your personality and your likely patterns of health. You can then choose actions that support wellness for someone of your personality type.

Patterns of personality also provide clues for wellness professionals to intervene in a way that is custom tailored for the needs of that individual, guiding the person toward a well state and even amplifying health, wellness, and peak performance through wellness counseling.

Quality of Life

The most obvious and desirable benefit of a well mind is a better quality of life, which of course is determined by each individual's model of the world. Our own viewpoint on reality, our own values and beliefs, will shape our definition of a great quality of life. A well person or family seeks to live consistently with their own definition of living well; so identifying the details of your desired outcomes makes it easier to tell when you're getting close.

Think about what a happy, satisfying, fulfilling life would be like, and pay attention to how you would need to be to have the best chance of creating that life for yourself. The more you act like the kind of person who would have the life you want, the more likely you'll do the things that kind of person would do, and that will lead to having those things in reality.

By noticing how you are already like this ideal version of you and by recognizing where you need to focus your energy to build the resources you need, you can grow into an enhanced version of yourself, more capable, and more attractive, which leads to a better quality of life, by your own definition.

Personal Growth

The end product of wellness psychology is ongoing personal growth. Rather than a psychological treatment for a mental or emotional condition, wellness psychology leads someone from wherever they are to wherever they want to go mentally and emotionally. Instead of stopping therapy when the symptoms resolve, wellness psychology is based on lifestyle choices and training in wellness habits that go far beyond "no symptoms" to a state of vitality and well-being. Being truly well has a vibration of self-esteem and *joie de vivre* that makes life seem more worth living, and the investment you make in your own education and development will come back to reward you many times over.

Spirituality

No discussion of wellness psychology would be complete without including the impact of spirituality on wellness. Higher beliefs and an appreciation of universal law form a foundation of wellness that is consistent with every spiritual tradition. Learning to balance physical, mental, emotional, and spiritual wellness is the ultimate objective of wellness psychology. (See *The Power of Full Engagement* by Jim Loehr and Tony Schwartz.)

Prosperity Consciousness

Einstein reputedly divided people in two groups —those who believe we live in a friendly universe and those who don't. Brilliant in its simplicity, it points out the fundamental basis of wellness psychology: that a well mind knows that we live in a friendly universe, brimming with opportunity and potential, awaiting our actions to trigger their manifestation.

A well mind sees abundance and realizes that there is enough so that each of us can have plenty. A well mind is aware of and utilizes the law of attraction, and understands how consistency with nature and makes sense and produces better overall results. Avoiding "lack thinking" and inappropriate, unnecessary pessimism conserves valuable energy and resources to invest in productive and gainful behaviors.

So, wellness psychology helps you become rich because a well mind is attractive, supple, creative, effective, capable, curious, motivated, and persistent.

Remember that being rich is not only a matter of money but a manifestation of inner wealth as well—rich relationships, rich appreciation for the splendor of natural living, and rich life experiences.

Positive expectancy and positive, powerful action toward a worthy goal creates the best probability of success and fulfillment. (See *The Dynamic Laws of Prosperity* by Catherine Ponder.)

Relationships and Family

While you can't be responsible for someone else's behaviors and values, you can help to create an environment that makes relationships work better. Gaining and maintaining rapport establishes a bond or connection that improves communication. Sharing and committing to support each other's values calms rocky waters and sets the stage for ongoing growth.

You can gain rapport by matching and mirroring someone—in other words, communicating in a similar style to make it comfortable for the other. By reflecting or matching their facial expression, voice tonality, body posture, word choice, or breathing pattern, you connect with the other person at a deep level.

Discussing values comes easier when you have rapport. Ask questions to find out what's important and why, so you can support the other person, and reasonably expect support in return. Make your needs and wants understood as well, so you can be supported in pursuing what is important to you.

Aging and Longevity

Well people enjoy their lives and want them to last as long as possible. That's why the wellness mindset usually accompanies other constructive, healthy lifestyle habits. By adopting positive behaviors like eating well, exercising, saying affirmations, and developing healthy self-talk, structuring a healthy system of values and beliefs, creating functional and fulfilling relationships, and balancing physical, mental, emotional, and spiritual energy, you build a foundation of wellness that preserves a well attitude, wellness-driven lifestyle choices, and an overall well experience in life.

You not only extend your life, you extend your quality of life deeper into later life. This is the ultimate objective of wellness psychology—to have the best life possible for as long as possible.

Three Challenges to Wellness

In the early twentieth century, D.D. Palmer wrote about disruptions in the brain and nervous system's control of body function known as subluxations. His intuition and his research agreed that there were three kinds of causes of such disturbances in body function, in essence, three challenges to wellness—trauma or injury, chemical toxicity or nutritional insufficiency, and autosuggestion or mental and emotional stress and dysfunction.

Wellness psychology, then, adds the component of mind care to the wellness equation that requires healthy structure and nervous system physiology, clean blood and body chemistry, and a mental and emotional environment that is conducive to happy and fulfilled living—in other words, the wellness lifestyle.

To learn more about wellness psychology, print out our recommended reading list at DiscoverWellnessCenter.com

13

Healthy Lifestyle Habits

In addition to the major components of wellness—alignment, exercise, nutrition, and healthy thinking—there are a number of other healthy habits that you can adopt to ensure that you are able to live your life of richness. These include minimizing the sugar in your diet, getting plenty of sleep, turning off the television, smoking cessation, attracting love and intimacy, and becoming an advanced citizen.

Smoking Cessation

Smoking throughout the day is akin to living inside a burning building. Smoking degrades the collagen of your skin, causing premature wrinkling, destroys the cells inside your lungs, and promotes heart disease, cataracts, and cancer because of the oxidizing radicals released into the blood stream. It can also contribute to back pain by dehydrating the spinal discs.

People stop smoking every day and so can you. Some people find acupuncture to be very helpful at reducing cravings, and many people have used nicotine patches for the same reason. But these are not as effective as your unswerving, absolute commitment to do whatever it takes to not smoke today. Just limit your not smoking to today only. You can tell yourself that you can have a cigarette tomorrow if you just make it through today. Tomorrow morning when you wake up, tell yourself the same thing. There are many addicts who have successfully kicked their alcohol, heroine, or cocaine addictions this way. Kicking any addiction is tough. You can expect to feel stressed, anxious, and irritable at first. To expect anything else is unreasonable. But you can also expect that over time it will become easier and easier to not smoke.

Stay Away from the Sugar!

In a recent study done by the USDA, it was reported that the average American consumes 134 pounds of refined sugar every year, or approximately 20 teaspoons of sugar per day. As hard as this may be to believe, consider the following facts:

- *A 12 oz. can of Pepsi® contains 10 teaspoons of sugar*
- *A 2 oz. package of candy contains 11 teaspoons of sugar*
- *A 16 oz. cup of lemonade contains 13 teaspoons of sugar*
- *A cup of Frosted Flakes® contains 4 teaspoons of sugar*

This high level of sugar intake is very unhealthy and contributes to obesity, Type 2 diabetes, heart disease due to elevated triglycerides, kidney stones, dental caries, chronic tiredness, and reactive hypoglycemia. Decreasing your sugar intake is as simple as avoiding foods that are high in refined sugars, such as soft drinks, candy, cake, and donuts, as well as most condiments. When you purchase sweetened food, look for products that are sweetened with apple juice or stevia, rather than sugar or high-fructose corn syrup.

Turn Off the Television

There are major trends in the health of both children and adults that have public health workers concerned: an increase in obesity and attention deficit disorder (ADD) and the amount of time spent watching television. Several recently published research studies indicate that television may be the culprit that leads to both of the others.

Watching television leads to obesity in two ways. First, every hour that you spend sitting in front of the television is an hour spent being inactive. Kids should be outside running around, riding bikes, and playing with their friends. Adults ought to be involved in hobbies and community activities. Sitting in front of the tube results in burning fewer calories and a reduction in overall metabolism. Also, a number of studies have shown that people who watch television simply eat more food.

Watching television also has detrimental effects on the brain's cognitive function, especially in kids. Studies published by the American Academy of Pediatrics have shown that children who watch more than two hours of television per day struggle more with aggressive behavioral problems, difficulty in concentrating, sleep disturbances, and a dramatically increased risk of alcohol consumption as teenagers. Although most studies have been conducted on children, other studies have shown that the results are just as valid for adolescents and adults as well. These negative effects can be explained by understanding the effect television has on the brain.

Broadcast television in the United States has a particular frequency of flicker that cannot be seen but which has an effect on brain function. A number of studies measured brain wave activity in people while they watch television. During these studies it was noticed that the brain waves in people watching television were similar to the brain waves of people who were in a trance. This trance-like state is associated with a decrease in the function of the cerebral cortex—the critical thinking part of the brain. When people are in this trance-like state for several hours per day, it becomes more difficult to focus their attention and control their impulses.

The American Academy of Pediatrics recommends that children watch no more than two hours of television per day— and it would be better to reduce this even further. Many health experts are now encouraging parents to completely eliminate watching television for children under the age of seven, to allow time for their brains to develop a bit more.

Pay Off Your Sleep Debt

Sleep expert and President of the American Sleep Research Institute Lynn Larson explains the link between sleep and decreased longevity is due to the immediate effect lack of sleep has on human performance. Missing sleep leads to poor decision making and affects everything we do: rushing when we should be methodical, forgetting important procedures, loss of attention (such as when driving), not having the energy to exercise, poorer reaction time, higher stress levels, elevated blood pressure, and inability to adapt to change. These things lead to accidents in the short term and poor health in the long term.

Research at ASRI suggests that the amount and quality of sleep we achieve has profound effects on wellness. Nightly sleep is critical for proper function of the brain, immune system, endocrine system, digestion, recovery from injury, and restoration of health. The lifestyle changes explained throughout this book are all intertwined with sleep. Sleep gives us the energy, the will, and the foundation to accomplish these changes.

Approximately 100 million Americans struggle with difficulty sleeping. If you have trouble falling asleep, or staying asleep, there are some "tricks" to improve the situation. To some extent, insomnia can be like the old expression about fear: there being nothing to fear but fear itself. Sometimes, just the fear of not being able to sleep causes enough stress to keep us awake. The guidelines that follow should help.

• *Don't look at the clock. Studies have shown that looking at the clock during the night increases insomnia. You will sleep more if you ignore the clock when you wake up during the night.*

• *Leave work at the office and don't take it to bed with you.*

• *If you wake during the night—do not think! Mental distraction is the name of the game. Try counting backwards from 100. The first times that you try this technique, you might count from 100 two or more times. It's OK. Eventually you will fall asleep at about 95. You are training yourself to stop thinking about problems and to fall asleep instead. It will take time to learn this good habit.*

• *No caffeine after dinner. The half-life of caffeine is about four hours.*

• *Alcohol makes you doze off quickly, but after it metabolizes it will interrupt sleep later in the night.*

Love and Intimacy

Although I have never seen a doctor write a prescription for daily doses of "love," bestselling authors such as Deepak Chopra, M.D., Bernie Siegal, M.D., and Dean Ornish, M.D., all write about the healing properties of love. Dr. Ornish says,

"Love may be the greatest of all disease-fighters, and it's about time doctors realized it." Dr. Ornish, a pioneer of wellness, has extensively researched how diet, exercise, and stress management can help reverse heart disease. His book *Love & Survival* explains that loneliness can kill you, while love and a sense of community can heal you.

Whether with a pet, a partner, or a spouse, sharing love is the most powerful force of nature. There is much concern that the smarter we get and the more technology we use, the lonelier we are and the more disconnected we feel. Dr. Ornish says that "the real epidemic isn't physical heart disease. It's spiritual heart disease: loneliness and isolation." Many experts agree.

It is amazing but true that the easiest thing in the world to do to improve our own health and wellness is to express our love for ourselves and for others. It doesn't cost anything and it doesn't have to take much time. The benefits of love are beyond measure.

Advanced Citizenry

Being an advanced citizen means that you dedicate some of your time, your thoughts, and your perspectives to some cause that you believe in. This may be something as simple as volunteering a few hours every month to visit with the senior citizens in the local nursing home, perhaps becoming a mentor to a child, or becoming active in your local government. Whatever it may be for you, by making your feelings known, you shape the world for future generations. Your ideas are more important than you may realize, so please participate in your local, state, and national organizations and add to the process with your own individual slant. The more that all of us do this, the more we'll develop a world about which we can all be proud.

Each of us has a sphere of influence, a circle of friends and acquaintances who need to hear our message. Whether you decide to do something small or great, please accept your share of the responsibility for moving our society ahead. If we all invest our own special something, the net effect will be a happy, healthy, and fulfilling life for us all.

How to Change Unhealthy Habits

There are three things that have to happen to successfully change a habit. The first is that you must make the decision to change. When you make a decision, you are affirming to yourself that you are willing to go to any lengths to make your wishes come true. This means that you will need to completely eliminate the word "try" from your vocabulary. When you say "I'll try to do my exercises," you are leaving an open door to not doing them. Then in your mind, if you don't do your exercises, that's okay because you only said you would "try" to do them. If you want to successfully change your habits to live a healthier life, you cannot leave an open door to your old habits. You need to just do it, just make a decision and not look back.

The second thing is to act "as if." Whenever you change what you are doing, it will feel unnatural. It may feel like you are doing something wrong, funny, or something that is just not you. In a way, you are right. When you change a habit, you are by definition acting in a way that is "just not you." But in a very short time, it will feel normal and it will seem strange that you ever acted any differently. Changing habits is like starting a new job: the first couple of weeks are stressful and disorienting, but if you just hang in there, you will feel at home before you know it.

The third is to work on yourself every day. The highest demonstration of a healthy self-image and self-esteem is the commitment to work on yourself each and every day. You experience an elevated consciousness when you realize your power to step up to your greatness or default to your weakness with every challenge, distraction, and decision. Working on yourself with consistency and persistence connects you to your inner wisdom and inner strength to become unstoppable.

14

Your Wellness Team

We live in an information-rich world. Are you aware that the amount of information doubles every two years? In today's world, cutting edge companies of all sizes are recruiting a Board of Directors to help them make more effective decisions and to increase their collective level of wisdom. Consulting with these wise individuals helps these organizations reduce the number of mistakes they make, as well as boost their organizational effectiveness.

Consistent with this concept, I have recruited a Board of Directors for my morning meditations, or as I like to call it, my "Hour of Power." I seek the wise counsel of many of history's greatest thinkers. This team concept gives me strength. It puts me on a proverbial all-star team with the best and the brightest. Of course all of the members of my Board of Directors don't actually get together with me to do my meditation and exercise routine; I simply think about what they would do in the circumstances I face in my life. Let me share some of the people who I have chosen to sit on my Board of Directors:

- *Albert Einstein for wisdom*
- *Mahatma Gandhi for leadership*
- *Mother Teresa for unconditional love*
- *Benjamin Franklin as an ideal statesman*
- *Bruce Lee for self-discipline*
- *The Dalai Lama for inner peace*
- *Oprah Winfrey for overcoming adversity*

As you get ready to assemble your own Board, first think about the qualities that made these men and women so admirable and how you would benefit from acquiring their qualities in your own life. Remember that the first step to realizing your life vision is defining it. The first step to becoming the person you want to become is to identify the characteristics and traits of your ideal version of your self.

The concept for the Board of Directors for building your character can be applied to wellness as well. My best friends from college and I always joked around whenever we would ask each other if we knew someone who could help us; we would always respond by saying "I've got a guy." Between the four of us someone always "had a guy" who could solve our car problems, real estate problems, financial problems, you name it. This is what you want to do for yourself by creating your own entourage of wellness care providers who can help you when you aren't feeling well and also help you promote your health when you are feeling your best.

Let me give you an example of what I mean by creating a team. Let's say for example that you go to your medical doctor complaining of neck pain. The doctor will ask you questions about how it happened, examine you, may prescribe pain relievers, anti-inflammatory medications, and muscle relaxants, and may refer you to a physical therapist. If after several weeks you do not get better, you go back to the medical doctor explaining that the pain does feel a little better when you take the medication, but the pain returns when the medication wears off. Not only that but you have difficulty working due to the side effects of the medication and you are starting to feel some numbness going into your shoulder and arm. The doctor will likely refer you to an orthopedist or neurologist for a consultation with a specialist.

You can see that it is the medical doctor who is the captain of the team that provides your medical needs. When you have an emergency, need medication, or require surgery to solve your problem, you go to see your medical doctor and the medical doctor directs you to the other specialists on the team; these might include nurses, physician's assistants, specialists, pharmacists, and many other players.

If, however, you are seeking a conservative drugless approach to healing or are seeking advice on how to improve your health and wellness, then you will find that the medical system is not designed to provide that type of care. So whom should you choose to be the captain of your wellness team?

Your wellness captain should be someone who has a high level of education in subjects such as anatomy and physiology, pathology, and wellness. It should be someone who understands what wellness means and understands how to create a wellness lifestyle. It should be someone who can help inspire you, keep you accountable, and provide you a variety of wellness resources, tools, and referrals to other great wellness specialists.

I truly believe that you want to choose a wellness chiropractor to be the captain of your wellness team—your Chief Wellness Officer, if you will. Let me explain why.

The Chief Wellness Officer

Chiropractors are licensed doctors with comparable education to medical doctors. The primary difference in education is that medical doctors spend more time studying subjects such as pharmacology, whereas chiropractors emphasize the study of the body's master system (the spine and nervous system), adjusting techniques, and nutrition.

Chiropractors are trained and experienced in knowing when to refer to medical doctors. Most people don't really want to take medication if there is a more conservative approach, but often people don't know where to go to find out what their problem is and, more importantly, are often afraid that it could be something really bad. So it seems like the right idea to go to the medical doctor to rule out the worst-case scenario. Often people are left unsatisfied because, although they may be able to rule out the worst, unless they need medication or surgery there is little else offered as a solution.

Chiropractors are trained to look for the cause of the problem by analyzing the spine and nervous system. After asking questions about your health history and examining your condition, they will be able to tell you whether you have a condition with which they can help or whether you have a condition that requires medicine or surgery. Chiropractors focus on correcting the cause of your problem, not just on suppressing your symptoms. Wouldn't it be best to start with the most conservative options first and then rely on medications or surgery if it's even necessary after giving the safer, less invasive approach a chance?

Chiropractors are covered by most health insurances and some drugless services such as manual therapy and therapeutic exercises may be covered by your health insurance when recommended by a chiropractor. This makes it more affordable and often more convenient to take care of yourself in a natural holistic manner.

Chiropractors are doctors trained with a holistic philosophy. The major premise of chiropractic is based on the recognition that there is intelligence in the universe. Chiropractors focus on ensuring that your body's own innate healing ability is working its best. By specializing in the care of your spine, which includes knowledge of the bones, muscles, and spinal cord, chiropractors influence the system that runs all other systems of your body. Only chiropractors provide a comprehensive solution to take care of the health of your spine and nervous system.

Chiropractors are usually more experienced with working with massage therapists, personal trainers, Pilates instructors, yoga teachers, nutritionists, homeopaths, naturopaths, acupuncturists, and other alternative medical providers. These are the players you want on your wellness team. You want a captain who knows what these providers do and who is able to help you decide when you need to use them. Most chiropractors have a working relationship with these types of providers, and they often work with them for their own personal wellness needs. The most recent trend for chiropractors is to run full service wellness centers offering you a convenient and affordable one-stop experience.

Some chiropractors have specialties in multiple wellness disciplines. For example Dr. Dick Versendaal teaches wellness professionals how to be Urgent Wellness Specialists using a protocol he developed over the past 50 years called Contact Reflex Analysis. It is a specialized healing technique analyzing multiple health factors including the reflexes of the body, along with eating, sleeping, working, smoking, drinking, and other lifestyle habits to determine someone's vitality. CRA provides practitioners an effective and efficient way to provide both chiropractic and nutritional care. CRA practitioners "perform precision adjustments and releases, enhance energy, nourish, build, support, and invigorate the body with the essence of life by integrating the activities of all parts of the body."

Another good reason for having your chiropractor be the leader of your wellness team is a very practical one based on my experience over the years. What I have seen is that many people with good habits slow down and sometimes have to stop exercising completely due to musculoskeletal pain. Many people come in to my office and tell me they have gained a lot of weight since not being able to workout due to their neck, back, or shoulder pain.

People say they get depressed because they want to be able to exercise but are afraid to—because their pain flares up when they begin exercising. If they had a wellness chiropractor, they would probably not have had to take so much time off from their routine and would likely have been able to resume exercising sooner.

How many times have you heard someone say they no longer play tennis, golf, run, ride horses, or engage in other physical activity because of their bad shoulder, knee, back, or neck? Often people have been to their doctor, have had x-rays and MRIs, tried physical therapy, lived on painkillers, and finally resigned themselves to the fact that they are "getting older." In some cases, the doctor says there is nothing more the person can do. When the doctor says this, however, what he or she often means is that there is nothing more the doctor can do. There is a difference.

There are many great wellness chiropractors in cities across America—it's just a matter of finding one. As I mentioned, not all chiropractors practice the same way. I recommend you interview several in order to find the one you like the best. When you call, you should ask if they offer complimentary consultations and even ask if they offer consultation by phone. Ask them to describe the type of practice they have. Ask them to describe their ideal client. Ask them their office hours and how long an average appointment should take. Ask them if they accept your health insurance, or if you don't have coverage, ask about what type of payment plans they have available. I recommend not basing your decision about which chiropractor to choose on whether or not your insurance covers it, and here's why: most people have a limited number of visits covered by their insurance and most people will require additional visits once their insurance benefits have been used. In some cases it may be more expensive to pay your co-payments only for the covered visits and full price once the insurance is exhausted.

I recommend that your comfort level with the doctor be your primary concern. Asking these questions is a great way to get to know the doctor; you will be able to make a better decision as to whether you like and trust him/her. Take the time to find someone who knows what she/he is talking about and who can provide you with great service.

To print a list of interview questions to ask your new wellness doctor
visit DiscoverWellnessCenter.com

Your Wellness Team

What I want you to do is to create an all-star wellness team. Seek out the best providers you can find, interview them, and make sure they can provide what you need to help create and support your wellness lifestyle.

The first step is to start asking people you know and trust if they know of any of the types of providers listed below. If they do, ask them questions about whom they see, why they see those providers, and whether they would recommend them. If you have friends who say that they like a practitioner, they like the experience and would recommend it, then that is a great place to start. You will be amazed at how many people you know who are already receiving wellness care.

Wellness Coach

Wellness coaches are like the nurses of wellness. They provide a vital role in helping people understand wellness, and most importantly are there to help you stay accountable to yourself. That's how you achieve results. Most of us do much better when we have help from someone knowledgeable.

Celebrities, athletes, executives, and the very wealthy are all people who have historically had the means to hire the help they need to get the results they want. But the growth of the coaching industry has made it affordable for just about everyone to be able to take advantage of the benefits of having a coach. Wellness coaches:

- *Assist people with identifying specific goals and then reaching those goals faster and with ease.*
- *Provide clients with the tools, perspective, and structure to accomplish a more thorough process of personal accountability.*

• *Reframe beliefs and create a point of focus upon which clients may reflect.*

The latest wellness trend is to have a wellness coach, someone who can help you by being an information resource and by inspiring you. If you really want to see results, remember that it is not a question of whether making healthy choices will benefit you. As long as you stay consistent with your healthy choices, you will always benefit. The longer you stick with those healthy habits, the better your health will be. It makes good sense to invest in hiring a coach who can help ensure you stay moving on the right track.

Massage Therapist / Body Worker

Massage is a system of pressing and kneading different soft tissues in the body (muscles, tendons, and ligaments). Massage offers a variety of health benefits: pain relief, relaxation, improved muscle tone, stimulation of circulatory and lymphatic systems, and more efficient elimination of waste throughout the body.

Although a single massage will reduce fatigue, relax you, and provide mild stress relief, the effects of massage are cumulative. A course of massage treatments will allow you to reap the most benefits. Ultimately, massage can rejuvenate you physically, mentally, and spiritually.

Massage rates can vary between $50 and $125 per hour, depending on the massage therapist and the location where you receive your massage. For example, you will pay more for someone to travel to your home to provide massage therapy. Fortunately, many chiropractic centers offer massage therapy as part of their services.

Personal Fitness Trainer

Another great way to get results is to make sure you are getting expert advice and supervision. A personal trainer is a great way to ensure that you are exercising safely and effectively to accomplish your goal. A personal fitness trainer is trained in developing and recommending exercise programs and often offers generally accepted nutritional advice as well. Personal trainers have a variety of certification programs. Peter Davis, CEO of IDEA Health & Fitness Association, the world's largest association for health and fitness professionals and InnerIDEA, an organization for mind/body professionals, feels that it is time for all wellness professionals to begin to work together as a team to look out for the best interest of their clients. The present fragmented wellness industry leaves the public confused. The most effective way for you to maximize your results is to work with certified trained professionals to ensure you are going to get maximum results safely.

You may look for a trainer who is a member of IDEA Health & Fitness Association at their Web site www.ideafit.com. Certifications include C.S.C.S. (Certified Strength and Conditioning Specialist) or a C.P.T. (Certified Personal Trainer). The most important thing is to find a trainer with whom you feel comfortable and with whom you would like to work. Knowing what to do is often the easy part; finding someone who will inspire you to stay with the program to get results is the hard part. Rates can range from $40-$90 per hour, and you can often receive discounts by purchasing packages of sessions.

Pilates Instructor

Pilates is a fast-growing trend in exercise. It helps strengthen core muscles and improves flexibility and strength for the entire body. One distinct advantage to some people is that Pilates exercises will not greatly increase muscle size.

Pilates, like yoga, focuses on a unique series of controlled and focused movements which engage both your body and mind. These exercises are performed on specially designed machines and are taught by trained instructors. There is very likely a Pilates studio near you. Alternatively, many fitness centers and health clubs offer Pilates classes which are open to the public. To learn more about Pilates, yoga, or other mind-body-spirit modalities, visit Inneridea.com.

Yoga Instructor

Yoga is another form of exercise that has become very popular. Yoga integrates mind, body, and spirit and enhances health in many ways. There are several types of yoga; whatever method is used, yoga incorporates specific postures and breathing exercises which are designed to enhance health and well-being.

There are many yoga studios to choose from in every major city. In addition, yoga classes may be taught at health clubs and even at community centers. Because of the variety of yoga methods, you may wish to take a few different classes to discover which is most comfortable and effective for you. Most centers offer an introduction to yoga for a reduced fee for those who simply wish take an initial class before signing up for a longer course.

Nutritionist

As you read in the chapter on nutrition, many different health concerns can be traced back to the foods we eat. Having a nutritionist or dietician can be a great resource. Nutritionists are professionals who can fully assess your condition, including lab testing for allergies and other health concerns. A dietician or nutritionist needs at least a bachelor's degree. Of the 46 states with laws governing dietetics, 31 require licensure. It's been my experience that as important as a nutritionist's education is, it is just as important to work with someone who inspires you to make the adjustments to your eating habits that will help you make lasting healthy changes.

Homeopath

Homeopathy is practiced by a wide variety of health care practitioners, including medical doctors, naturopathic physicians, nurse practitioners, dentists, chiropractors, acupuncturists, and others. There are also professional homeopaths who practice only homeopathy and are unlicensed in any other discipline. You will find a variety of homeopathic remedies at most health food stores, and these can often be an effective way of relieving symptoms without the use of pharmaceuticals.

Homeopathy is a system of healing based on three core principles:

1. Like cures like
2. Minimal dose
3. Single remedy

Homeopaths will often recommend a single "remedy" that is an extremely diluted product of something that would produce a similar symptom in a healthy person. There are 300 major remedies, with up to 3000 from which homeopaths can choose to treat specific conditions.

Naturopath

A licensed naturopathic physician attends a four-year naturopathic medical school. Naturopaths are educated in all of the same basic sciences as medical doctors, and in addition to that education, the naturopath is also required to complete four years of training in clinical nutrition, acupuncture, homeopathic medicine, botanical medicine, psychology, and counseling.

Naturopaths study holistic and nontoxic approaches to therapy and strongly emphasize disease prevention and optimizing wellness. As with medical doctors, naturopathic physicians must pass rigorous professional licensing exams, and are fully qualified to be primary care general practice physicians.

Acupuncturist

Acupuncture encourages the body to promote natural healing and improve function. Acupuncture involves inserting tiny sterilized, stainless-steel needles into specific points on the body—just barely through the surface of the skin. Stimulating these points causes biochemical and physiological changes which can help treat a wide variety of illnesses.

Dentist

The dental profession has done an exceptional job teaching people about wellness. Although some people do not go to the dentist until they are in pain, few people dispute that it is a good idea to see your dentist for preventative care and optimal hygiene.

An Exercise Buddy

I highly recommend that you have a buddy. Besides the obvious benefits of friendship, an exercise buddy helps you to stay consistent by ensuring that you have a good time with someone you like, who also wants to make exercise part of a healthy lifestyle. This can help a lot when the weather isn't great or you don't really feel like going to exercise, but you know that your buddy will be there and ask why you didn't show up. We have all experienced not wanting to work out, but sometimes you will show up anyway because you have a buddy you don't want to let down.

Summary

First, find a great wellness chiropractor you like and who you feel confident can help you. If at first you don't succeed, keep on interviewing chiropractors until you find one with whom you do feel comfortable.

Explain that you are putting together your all-star wellness team and you would like his or her help. Then you should be able to get started. Ask if your chiropractor offers additional wellness services. If not, ask your employer if wellness coaching is offered as part of an employee wellness program

Start building your team by following up on the referrals you receive from your wellness chiropractor, your wellness coach, and your friends. This will be the most efficient and most effective way of building your wellness team. It is great to work with practitioners who work with each other.

To print a Wellness Team Worksheet, please visit

DiscoverWellnessCenter.com.

15

Wellness Essentials

The purpose of this chapter is to provide you with a resource for finding additional information and products that will help you live a healthier life. Use this as your personal wellness product guide. You can find out more information about all of these products on our Web site, DiscoverWellnessCenter.com. If you have a favorite product that is not listed here, please let me know.

I always do my very best to stay current with the latest and greatest wellness products on the market. I recommend you consult your wellness chiropractor or specialist to determine which of the following products best fits your needs and supports your goals. In addition to their expertise and service, often they offer these products at their wellness centers for your convenience.

Alignment

As I discussed in chapter 9, maintaining proper alignment throughout the day is very important for your health. The following products are specially designed to help you maintain a healthy curve in your neck and back. Like brushing your teeth for a few minutes every day, using these tools for a few minutes each day can help improve your posture and reduce your risk for cervical degeneration by improving your cervical curve. This will help to offset the daily stress most people put on their neck by sitting at a desk or in front of their computers all day, or by sitting in traffic and driving with poor posture, which often leads to the condition referred to as FHP, Forward Head Posture.

Cervical Curve Devices

Depending on your age and condition of your spine, your wellness doctor may recommend you use tools to help reduce spinal degeneration due to long-term spinal misalignment. Devices such as a Posture Pump, Cervical Roll, Spinal Fulcrum, Spinal Traction, and The Posture Right™ by Neck Orthotic can help reduce spinal decay and in many cases actually increase the health of your spine by helping restore the natural curves of your spine. Restoring the natural curves of your spine helps to maintain proper nutrition to your discs, and improves your posture and range of motion. People regularly report that these types of tools help reduce pain and increase mobility.

Experts suggest that x-ray examinations indicate that proper alignment of the spine helps to reduce the rate of spinal degeneration, which can have a variety of overall positive health benefits. In addition, we have all seen what people whose posture worsens with aging look like; there is little that can be done to improve posture once decades of damage and neglect have set in. Now is the time to begin to care for your spine.

Cervical Pillow

There are a variety of different types of pillows made of different grades of foam, which have custom curves designed into them to support your neck. If you are like most people, you sleep on your pillow for six to nine hours every night. Shouldn't you sleep on something that will help you maintain your good health, not something that will slowly allow your posture to get worse and worse over the years?

☙ Discover Wellness Recommends

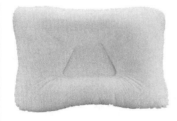

Cervical pillows are a simple way to reduce stress on the neck and upper back. Core Products is a leading producer of cervical pillows, lumbar supports, and other products that help the body maintain healthy alignment.

Lumbar Support

A support for your low back is essential to have in the chairs in which you will spend most of your time. Most furniture companies do not manufacture chairs that are actually healthy for you. The seats are often hard, rather than cushioned, and the position of your spine is often very poor and sometimes even damaging. Think of having a lumbar support for your office chair, your car seat, and your favorite reading chair at home.

One idea is to have a lumbar support that you can take with you when you travel on airlines. Someday I hope to see airlines provide lumbar supports for people the way they do blankets and pillows. Why not ask the flight attendants next time you are on a flight? Tell them your chiropractor said it would make the flight much more enjoyable and less damaging to your health. If enough people ask for it, perhaps one day they will get the hint.

Another tool to help keep healthy alignment includes a special shaped support pillow that rests between your legs while you are lying on your side. The Leg Spacer® is designed to align your lower extremities in order to relieve pressure on your low back, hips, and knees. It is very comfortable to sleep with, and once again not only helps reduce pressure on your low back but also helps you get a better night's sleep.

I also like the Back Vitalizer™ very much. This is a rectangular air-filled low back pillow that you either use behind your low back, or as a seat cushion. The product helps enhance the hydration of spinal discs, improves muscle blood circulation, and helps to reduce pain while you are sitting. It also simulates the effect of sitting on an exercise ball in that it activates your core muscles in order to stabilize your pelvis on the air pocket. Because of its simple design you can use it at work or at home, take it to sporting events, use it in your car, and bring it on an airplane. The Back Vitalizer™ is extremely helpful for people who sit a lot, and it feels remarkably comfortable.

Ergonomic Work Station

If you are like many people, you spend almost half of all of your waking hours sitting at a desk. It is therefore important that your chair, desk and other equipment help your body maintain good posture and alignment. A healthy work station must include proper seating, adjustable keyboard and mouse, an adjustable computer monitor position, lighting, and proper positioning of your work. These are all critical to minimize the stress on your body. An improper chair position, cradling the phone between your ear and shoulder, or straining your neck to look at your computer monitor is not a big deal every once in a while; but when you do the same repetitive motions for several hours a day, several days a week, several weeks a month, and so on, you find that your body eventually has to give and in many cases will suffer pain, discomfort, poor posture, and spinal disc damage. Unfortunately, most people don't correlate these problems to their day-to-day activity because they think these problems have to be caused by a specific traumatic event. That's just not the case.

Desk Chair

The basics of a healthy ergonomic workstation include a biomechanically correct chair to sit in. It is best if it is adjustable to support your unique height and curves. HumanScale™ offers a variety of seating options designed to keep you healthy and well while you are working. Choose from a variety of models including the Freedom™ or Liberty™. Not only do they support your spine and adjust to offer a perfect fit for your body to work in, they also feature beautiful, award-winning designs. You will notice them on the sets of many of today's most popular television shows. These products are an investment in your health if you sit at your desk often.

A great new cost-effective desk chair is an exercise ball that sits on a stand, such as the Ball Chair by Gaiam®. These are terrific and very affordable. These chairs actually help you strengthen your core muscles while sitting on them. It's like a workout while you're working.

🍎 Discover Wellness Recommends

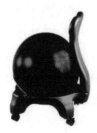

Sitting in a desk chair all day leads to weakness of the muscles that help to stabilize the low back. This contributes to increased low back pain, stiffness, and susceptibility to injury. Gaiam® has developed the perfect solution: the Ball Chair. Sitting on a Ball Chair is a simple way to keep your body properly aligned and maintain strong, healthy, low back support muscles.

Monitor Arm

First it was great when computer monitors went from taking up so much desk space to the new flat panels, but they are still on the desk taking up space and don't have too many ways to adjust their position to best fit a person's work station. HumanScale™, a leader in ergonomic office furniture, offers a variety of computer monitor arms that can get your monitor off your desk. Monitor arms are completely adjustable, so that you can see your monitor where you want to, when you want to. It's a brilliant idea whose time has come.

Headsets

If you talk on the phone regularly and for long periods of time, a headset is a great tool to prevent headaches, stiff necks, and sore shoulders. If you really want a new and healthy experience, invest in a cordless headset. Being able to stand up, walk around, and use your hands while talking on the phone is not only healthier, it helps you be more productive. One of the most popular brands is Plantronics®.

Keyboard / Mouse Wrist Pads

Many computer keyboards now include wrist pads as standard accessories. There are, however, ways to upgrade and enjoy the benefits of a liquid-filled or foam pad designed to comfortably support your wrists while typing and using your mouse. If you use a computer regularly, these are worth the investment.

One of the more innovative ideas that has recently been invented is a washable keyboard and mouse. This is helpful for families with kids and in high traffic areas such as hospitals, schools and businesses. Look for Unotron's Spill-Seal® washable keyboards and Scroll-Seal® washable mouse.

Orthotics

Your feet are the base that your body stands on. If your feet are weak or have structural problems, this can lead to problems in your knees, hips, and low back and can even cause headaches. Many people wear orthotics because they are good for their feet, but orthotics are even more important for those who experience pain after extended walking or standing.

The most popular brand of orthotics is Foot Levelers. Foot Levelers, Inc. has been in business for over 50 years. When you order orthotics, a cast or mold will be made of each of your soles. Some doctors have started to use high tech digital scanners. At least 16 different measurements of your feet are taken to ensure that your feet, and therefore your foundation, are more firmly supported.

Please note that the orthotics and insoles that you buy at your drug store are not the same as the high quality orthotics that you can have custom made, even though they look similar. Insoles may effectively reduce pressure by increasing the padding under your feet, but orthotics are customized and

---

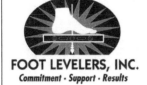

Discover Wellness Recommends

FOOT LEVELERS, INC.
Commitment · Support · Results

Your feet are the foundation of your body, supporting you when you stand, walk, or run. It's important to understand that all Foot Levelers Spinal Pelvic Stabilizers are custom-made to support all three arches of the foot, which creates a balanced foundation. That means that no matter which Stabilizer you choose, you'll get optimal results.

---

provide a foot bed that is molded specifically for each of your feet based on their unique shape and size. Customized orthotics are also a worthy investment. Ask your wellness chiropractor whether Foot Levelers custom orthotics are appropriate for you.

Buy Good Shoes

Most people spend close to two-thirds of their life in shoes, so finding proper fitting shoes is very important. Feet endure tremendous pressures of daily living. An average day of walking brings a force equal to several hundred tons on your feet. Feet are subject to more injury than any other part of the body, underscoring the need to protect them with proper shoes. Here is a quick guide to selecting the right shoes for your feet.

- *Always have your feet measured while you're standing.*
- *Always try on both shoes, and walk around the store.*

- *Always buy for the larger foot; feet are seldom precisely the same size.*
- *Don't buy shoes that need a 'break-in' period; shoes should be comfortable immediately.*
- *Don't rely on the size of your last pair of shoes; your feet do get larger.*
- *Shop for shoes later in the day, as feet tend to swell during the day.*
- *Select a shoe with a leather upper, stiff heel counter, good cushioning, and flexibility at the ball of the foot.*
- *Try on shoes while you're wearing the same type of socks or stockings you expect to wear with the shoes.*
- *If you wear prescription orthotics, you should take them along to shoe fittings.*

Sleep on a Good Mattress

Most people spend approximately one-third of their entire life lying in bed. The quality of your mattress can make a huge difference between waking up feeling refreshed and waking up in pain. In fact, old worn-out mattresses are an extremely common contributor to chronic back and neck pain.

Good health and sleep are closely linked. Just as we improve our eating habits for better health, we should also improve our sleep habits. Good sleep not only reduces back problems, it also helps to prepare us for a more productive day. If you think that your mattress may be past its prime, here are some tips to help you select the right mattress for you:

- *There is no single mattress that works well for all people. Look for a mattress that is adjustable in firmness and support.*

- *Find a mattress that has proper support for good sleep posture. Good sleep posture is nearly the same as good standing posture, with the ear, shoulder, hip, and ankle all in alignment. This will require different levels of support for different parts of the body.*

- *Know when it's time to get a new mattress. If an old mattress sags visibly in the middle, it is definitely time to purchase a new one.*

- *Shop for the best value and quality of the mattress rather than for price. A high-quality mattress is usually worth the investment, considering the effect a mattress can have on your overall health and comfort.*

- *Give the mattress a test-run in your home. When shopping, many people spend only a few minutes on a mattress in a showroom. They usually spend more time checking the comfort of a couch! It is not possible to determine if a mattress is right for you unless you sleep on it.*

Back Saver Wallet™

Most men carry a wallet in their back pockets and in many cases it can be over a half an inch thick. Sitting on a half-inch wedge for hours at a time over a period of years is one of the most overlooked causes of spinal misalignments and spinal pain including back pain, neck pain, and even headaches. My recommendation is to clean out your wallet and carry only what is really necessary.

An innovative new product that has a unique patented design and can reduce the size of your wallet by over 50 percent is called the TPK® Back Saver Wallet™; I like to think of it as the "wellness wallet." Its unique thin design allows for it to be carried in your front pocket instead of your back pocket, restoring the natural tripod effect of your spine when you are seated. You'll be amazed at what a difference it makes.

Healthy Back Pack

Another important wellness essential product is an ergonomically designed backpack. It is amazing that we can put thousands of pages of data onto a microchip smaller than the eye can see, yet kids are carrying backpacks that are heavier than ever filled with text books. Many schools are taking away kids' lockers, making the problem even worse. Some kids carry backpacks with up to 40 percent of their body weight or more.

You can see them walking to school leaning forward to offset the weight on their backs.

Until schools figure out a way to make the loads lighter, we recommend that you get a backpack that is designed to help your child stand up straighter. A favorite is the AirPack® Backpack designed by Core Products because of its patented shoulder straps and inflatable lumbar cushion which, when properly adjusted, redistributes the weight from the shoulders and upper back into the hips, promoting a healthier upright standing posture.

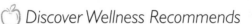

Discover Wellness Recommends

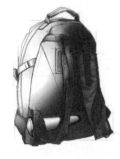

Most backpacks are designed for appearance, rather than for health. Consequently, many children are injured each year by backpacks that do not distribute the weight of their books properly. Core Products offers a revolutionary design in backpacks called the AirPack®. The AirPack® helps to reduce the risk of back injury from carrying heavy books.

Exercise

There is a tremendous variety of products on the market designed to help you exercise more effectively and efficiently. Listed next are some of the most important products that you should consider:

Exercise Ball

These days an exercise ball is a great tool to have and use at home. You can do a thorough workout on it, you can stretch on it and you can use it as a desk chair. Make sure to get the correct size. There are great videos that you can use to learn basic exercise routines.

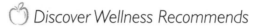 Discover Wellness Recommends

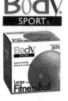

Fitness balls are simple, yet highly effective tools for maintaining good health. They are great for stretching and allow you to perform a wide variety of low-impact exercises that will improve your muscle strength, coordination, and balance. Body Sport is a leading manufacturer of high-quality exercise balls.

Resistance Bands / Weights

In order to keep your muscles strong, you must stress them by resistance training. Dumbbell weights or resistance bands are great ways to strengthen your muscles. Resistance bands are great because they are easy to travel with. Take them on your next business trip and you won't miss a workout wherever you are. Thera-Band® is an industry-leading producer of high quality resistance band home exercise products.

BOSU®

A great way to work on strengthening the core muscles that wrap around your waist and support your spine, as well as to improve your balance and coordination, is to use a new workout tool called a BOSU®, which stands for "both sides up." On one side, it is a half of a balance ball; on the other side it is a flat surface. This is a great tool that allows you to complete a variety of different workouts. This is a great way to reduce your risk of injury as you age. Many age-related injuries are due to falls because of poor balance and coordination.

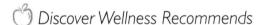 Discover Wellness Recommends

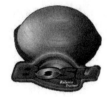 *BOSU® is a simple, safe, and inexpensive workout tool that is very effective at improving balance and strength in the core muscles of the body.*

Instructional Videos, Books, and Online Resources

With today's technology there really is no good excuse not to stretch and exercise properly. You can check out exercise videos for free at the local library, rent them from video stores, or access free information online. You can even purchase exercise, yoga, and Pilates programs to download onto your iPod®. An excellent series of instructional videos is avaliable from Gaiam.com.

Foam Roll

A foam roll is exactly what it sounds like: a long roll made of foam which can be used to help with balance and coordination exercise, to help you stretch your muscles, and to "roll out" the stress and tension in your muscles, in order to release the lactic acid that builds up in muscles and causes pain.

Core Trainer

The Core Trainer is an innovative, effective piece of exercise equipment from Panasonic that allows you to sit down and perform low impact exercises that help lead to high impact results. This is made possible by innovative "counter-balance exercise technology," which constantly moves you off your center of balance, forcing you to use your thigh, back, stomach, and other core muscles to re-gain your balance. This reaction efficiently and effectively maximizes the building of core body strength while minimizing body and joint stress.

 Discover Wellness Recommends

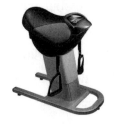

The Core Trainer by Panasonic is an effective tool for maximizing the strength and stability of the body's core muscles around the abdomen and low back; effectively reducing the risk of injury and maximizing health.

Power Plate™

The Power Plate™ is an innovative piece of equipment that employs Advanced Vibration Technology™ to achieve a higher level of fitness faster than than traditional training. The vibrations of the Power Plate™ causes rapid involuntary muscular contractions, which results in an increased workout intensity with no additional effort. The Power Plate™ is used by many professional athletes who seek the most efficient and effective fitness tools. My personal trainer had me use the Power Plate™ as part of my training and I loved it.

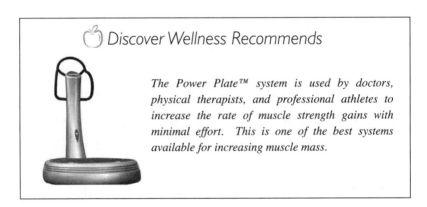

🍎 Discover Wellness Recommends

The Power Plate™ system is used by doctors, physical therapists, and professional athletes to increase the rate of muscle strength gains with minimal effort. This is one of the best systems available for increasing muscle mass.

Biometrics

There are a variety of different tools you can now purchase for a reasonable cost to help you better understand how your body functions in different environments. You will learn more about yourself and improve your results by measuring your progress. The basic tool most people are already familiar with is the scale to measure your weight.

There are also affordable ways to measure your own body mass index (BMI), your blood pressure, and your heart rate. Heart rate monitors are a great way to watch how your heart responds to exercise so that you can modify your exercise routine to accomplish more specific goals or track your improvement in fitness level.

Another simple tool to measure your progress is an inexpensive pedometer. A pedometer measures the number of steps you take. See if you can begin to make walking 10,000 steps per day a habit for life.

Wrist Metabolism Monitor

If you are a gadget junkie, a professional athlete, or just like to have the most advanced new technology, you'll want the Suunto T6. It is a wristwatch that measures a variety of statistics while you workout, such as heart rate, oxygen consumption, and respiratory rate. You can then wirelessly upload your data to your computer to track your progress. There are even programs that will correlate your data with sport-specific training programs. You have to check this out. It's cutting edge technology that can help you get better results, faster.

Nutritional Supplements

One easy change to make as you improve your eating habits is to buy organic food. It is important to purchase organic produce that is fresh and local, and meat that is free of antibiotics and hormones. Reducing the amount of pesticides and other chemicals in your diet reduces your risk of cancer and other diseases related to toxins used in the agricultural industry. In addition, the water used to produce organic food is cleaner, the soil is healthier, and the animals are usually raised more humanely.

Essential Fatty Acids

One component of nutrition that deserves significant attention is essential fatty acids (EFAs). EFAs cannot be produced by the body and therefore must come from the food we eat. They are the main structural components of our cell membranes, and keep our cell walls healthy by allowing nutrients to flow in and toxins to flow out. The three main essential fatty acids are omega-3, omega-6, and omega-9. Most people consume enough omega-6 and omega-9 fatty acids in the form of vegetable oils. However, we are often deficient in omega-3 fatty acids that come from foods such as flax seed, fish, and borage oil. Omega-3 fatty acids are known to help with cardiovascular, joint, and skin health, and to improve mood. Supplementing daily with an EFA capsule or liquid oil is essential to properly nourish your body.

Vitamin Supplements

Unless you live on an organic farm, most experts agree that you should take a daily supplement in order to ensure that your body is receiving the nutrients necessary to promote your optimum health. Multivitamin supplements help your body stay nourished to keep healthy and strong. One of my favorite products is the NutriWell Pack formulated by Biotics Research. Besides being a high-quality blend of basic wellness nutrients formulated by scientists, doses are conveniently packaged in individual daypacks, eliminating the need for multiple bottles and pill counting. Also, they are easy to take with you on the go or on a trip.

Greens

Dietary essentials for wellness include getting the five to ten servings of vegetables and fruits per day that will provide you with antioxidants, fiber, vitamins, and minerals necessary for optimum functioning at the cellular level. To help you achieve this goal, I suggest a whole food phytonutrient blend, often called "green powder." Of course, please remember it is best for you to eat real fruits and vegetables.

Protein

Protein is another nutritional foundation essential to building and maintaining muscle during every stage of life.

Protein provides a number of benefits in the areas of weight management, immune support, and bone health. As you know, it is always best to nourish your body with natural organic foods, but you may also benefit by adding a protein powder to your supplement routine. This is recommended especially for people who are on vegetarian diets, the elderly, and those striving for maximum energy.

Detoxification Products

Every person should cleanse the system of toxins and let the digestive tract rest at least once each year. Cleansing is one of the most direct and effective ways to improve your overall health quickly. Free radicals and toxins can build up in your body over time and may cause fatigue, poor immune function, sleep disturbances, aches, pains, and low energy. There are cleansing programs and supplements available that help the body repair and remove toxins. It is generally recommended that you contact a nutrition professional when choosing a detoxification program.

Relaxation

In the past couple of decades there has been a lot of fascinating research into the connection between the mind and the body. Your emotions and your mood have a tremendous impact on your physical state. As discussed in previous chapters, people who are stressed suffer from disturbed sleep and suppressed immune function, as well as an increased risk of heart disease, depression, high blood pressure, and cognitive impairment. Reducing your stress by following the suggestions made in chapter 12 will improve your health and quality of life. Here are some additional products that can help you.

Relaxation Audios

There are many styles of relaxation audios. Some people like listening to chanting; some like guided visualizations, some like male voices, while others prefer female voices, some like sounds of nature. Try different styles and experience how they make you feel. The most important part about relaxation is that it becomes a routine. Whatever your personal preference, you should make it a habit.

Get creative and build your own relaxation station. Choose a quiet place, include your favorite calming aromatherapy, a candle, and something comfortable to sit on that allows you

---

Discover Wellness Recommends

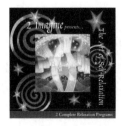

Relaxation products from 2Imagine are designed to bypass conscious awareness without the use of subliminal messages. These suggestions are completely audible, yet subtly embedded by using the words and phrases of the metaphors themselves to facilitate relaxation.

to effortlessly sit in a healthy posture. Sit in silence, listen to calming music, or enjoy a guided meditation. It's all about relaxing your mind and body, rejuvenating, and reconnecting with your self.

Home Massage

Home massage pads and recliners are not just for the rich and famous. There are a variety of home massage systems that you can use over your favorite chair at home, or you can replace that old recliner with a new healthy way to sit back and enjoy your favorite room in the house. Many wellness centers use massage chairs in their reception area. Try one and you'll instantly feel more relaxed and at ease.

Pain-Relieving Topicals

Sometimes your body could use some heat or cold to help it relax. Topical creams such as BioFreeze® and Prossage™ help to relieve muscle aches and soreness. BioFreeze® contains

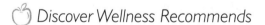

Discover Wellness Recommends

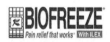

BioFreeze® products contain ILEX, an herbal extract from a South American holly shrub. ILEX is used around the world in various health and wellness formulations. BioFreeze® topical analgesic does not use waxes, oils, aloe, or petroleum. The result is a fast-acting, penetrating, long-lasting pain reliever.

ILEX, an herbal extract from a South American holly shrub. BioFreeze® is used by thousands of doctors to provide people simple, effective, temporary pain relief as an adjunct to their care.

Hot and Cold Packs

Cold therapy works by constricting blood vessels, resulting in a decrease of blood flow to the affected area, thereby reducing painful swelling. The risk of cold therapy is freezing the skin. To avoid this, simply make sure that there is at least one layer of clothing between your skin and the ice pack itself. Some doctors recommend using the R.I.C.E. method, which stands for Rest, Ice, Compression, and Elevation, to help reduce swelling for the first 72 hours following an injury, such as minor strains and sprains. As with all injuries, you will want to consult with your wellness chiropractor to ensure to that your spine and joints are properly aligned.

Heat therapy works by opening blood vessels, causing an increase in blood flow to the area of application. This helps to relax muscles and decrease pain. Heat therapy is recommended for chronic muscle stiffness and soreness. Apply a warm pack to the affected area for 20 minutes followed by 20 minutes of rest with no heat. Check your skin frequently to make sure that you are not getting too hot. Remember to always consult your health care provider regarding any type of home treatment.

There are several different types of hot and cold packs. Discover Wellness recommends the Core Products' Dual

Comfort Therapy Packs. These packs offer the benefits of both heat and cold in one pack. You can store the packs in the freezer to have ready as a cold pack, or take directly from the freezer to the microwave to use as a heating pad. The Dual Comfort packs also provide two different surfaces one providing "rapid release" therapy and one providing "slow release" therapy. Remember to always follow the directions of your health care provider regarding any treatment of injury.

Q-Link™

One of my favorite tools to help feel more energy, less stress, greater focus and overall improved well-being is the Q-Link™. The Q-Link™ is a pendant you wear around your neck which acts like a tuning fork for your body's "biofield," allowing your body to function at its optimum state. When we encounter a world of various energetic frequencies from things like cell phones, computer monitors, televisions, and more, our energy is affected. Q-Link™ products help to ground our energy by reversing the process allowing us to feel a greater sense of ease and relaxation. Q-Link™ products are particularly popular with people who require focus and concentration—especially golfers, who notice substantial improvements to their game. Many PGA players wear the Q-Link™, and there is a substantial amount of research to prove why it works. Q-Link™ technology also is available in a clock radio and a unit that can ground an entire room.

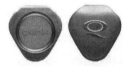

🍎 *Discover Wellness Recommends*

When you wear the Q-Link™ Pendant, your body's energy becomes more refined, clarified, and strengthened. So when you are under stress, you can cope more effectively.

Earthing Technology

Earthing is the deliberate use of the earth's free electrons and naturally occurring frequencies to support body recovery. Science has shown it increases relaxation, reduces stress, promotes sleep, helps normalize hormone levels, and reduces pain. The incredible benefits from the earthing technology come from sleeping on a special patented cotton bed sheet. That's all there is to it. Just do what you do normally.

Lance Armstrong and his team used the earthing technology during the last three Tour de France victories. The riders slept better, had less pain, and recovered more fully than their competitors, which gave the team a competitive advantage. James Oschman, Ph.D., author of *Energy Medicine: The Scientific Basis*, has said that "earthing has to be the most profound health discovery of our time."

StressEraser™

A new tool I found and like a lot is called the StressEraser™. It is an iPod®-looking, handheld biofeedback device that helps you focus on your breathing and scores you based on how well you relax. It is sort of like a video game to erase your stress. If you like technology and want a tool to help you focus on your breathing, this is a great solution. They say that if you use it for fifteen minutes before you go to sleep at night, you will feel less stressed, better rested, and overall much healthier. They are right.

Day Spa

Making time to take care of yourself is the common theme of wellness. Day spas are becoming more and more popular. They also make great gifts and employee incentives, because many people just aren't willing to spend the money on themselves. Check out a day spa near you; go for a relaxing facial, manicure, and pedicure. Perhaps you would prefer a massage and hot tub. Day spas are great ways to take a mini-vacation for yourself without the travel. You will feel rested, rejuvenated, and look your best.

Resort Spas, Vacation Retreats
and Seminars

When a day at the spa just isn't enough and you have some time to travel, why not travel to a destination resort and spa? Great ones include The Claremont Resort & Spa, Miraval, Canyon Ranch, and The Chopra Center at LaCosta Resort and Spa.

Cruises are great ways to enjoy wellness vacations. Just make sure you choose one that promotes wellness, so you don't actually lose progress by eating your way from island to island. Many of these great resorts, spas, and cruises offer incredible packages that include seminars and workshops with bestselling authors and wellness experts.

Additional Recommended Products
for Your Health

It is essential these days to ensure that you are drinking not only an adequate amount of water every day, but also to make sure that you are drinking clean purified filtered water. A home water filter can help you save thousands of dollars on bottled water. It is more convenient and friendlier to the environment by reducing the need for so many little plastic bottles.

An air purifier helps to make sure you filter the air inside your home or office. With so many pollutants in the atmosphere, it is best for your health to do what you can to reduce your exposure to toxins in the areas you spend the most time. It makes taking a nice deep breath that much healthier for you.

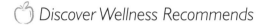 Discover Wellness Recommends

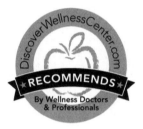

For a complete list of all products that
Discover Wellness recommends, please visit:
DiscoverWellnessCenter.com

16

Staying Healthy Can Make You Rich!

C onsider for a moment what a difference it would make in your financial life if you had an extra $1,000, $2,000, or even more per month available to put into your savings account or to invest. According to a study published in the journal *Health Affairs*, the average health care cost per American—every man, woman, and child in the United States —is $6,280.[2]

If we all just made a few simple changes in our lives, such as getting more exercise, eating better, keeping our spine in proper alignment, and eliminating some of our bad habits, we could dramatically reduce the stress on our health care system.

So, let's do some math and prove how, in fact, staying healthy can make you rich. If you start with the amount reported by the study previously cited above, every man, woman, and child in the United States is spending $6,280 per year. That's over $25,000 for a family of four. This may be a new way of thinking about how much health care costs us, but one way or the other we are all paying for it through higher prices and higher taxes—even those who are not sick are paying their share. Most studies conservatively suggest that improving your lifestyle habits can decrease your risk of disease by at least 50 percent, and most experts agree that if you improve multiple lifestyle habits, you can reduce your risk of disease by much more. It should not be hard to believe that a family of four can save over $1,000 per month.

Let's see how much each and every American could save if we were to use the conservative estimate that making at least one, if not several, lifestyle habit improvements can reduce our risk of disease by 50 percent. Reducing $6,280 by 50 percent equals $3,140 per person in annual savings. Let's assume that the cost of health care continues to rise at a conservative estimate of eight percent per year.

$6,280 x 4 = $25,120   *Present cost of health care for a family of four*

$25,120 ÷ 2 = $12,560   *50 percent savings due to wellness lifestyle*

$12,560 ÷ 12 = $1,047   *Monthly savings to invest*

A healthy 30 year old who stays well and adopts healthy habits can theoretically save over $1 million by the time she is 65 years old. I say theoretically because we are dealing with averages for all Americans. This is money spent in a variety of ways, as mentioned, through increased prices, increased taxes,

How Staying Healthy Can Make You Rich

Total Health Care Costs

Per Capita Cost of Health Care Reduced by 50%

Year	Beginning Value	6% Growth	Amount Saved Inflated @ 8%	Ending Value
1	$0	$0	$3,140	$3,140
2	$3,140	$188	$3,391	$6,720
3	$6,720	$403	$3,662	$10,785
4	$10,785	$647	$3,955	$15,388
5	$15,388	$923	$4,272	$20,583
6	$20,583	$1,235	$4,614	$26,432
7	$26,432	$1,586	$4,983	$33,000
8	$33,000	$1,980	$5,381	$40,362
9	$40,362	$2,422	$5,812	$48,596
10	$48,596	$2,916	$6,277	$57,788
11	$57,788	$3,467	$6,779	$68,034
12	$68,034	$4,082	$7,321	$79,438
13	$79,438	$4,766	$7,907	$92,111
14	$92,111	$5,527	$8,540	$106,177
15	$106,177	$6,371	$9,223	$121,771
16	$121,771	$7,306	$9,961	$139,038
17	$139,038	$8,342	$10,757	$158,138
18	$158,138	$9,488	$11,618	$179,244
19	$179,244	$10,755	$12,548	$202,546
20	$202,546	$12,153	$13,551	$228,250
21	$228,250	$13,695	$14,635	$256,580
22	$256,580	$15,395	$15,806	$287,781
23	$287,781	$17,267	$17,071	$322,119
24	$322,119	$19,327	$18,436	$359,883
25	$359,883	$21,593	$19,911	$401,387
26	$401,387	$24,083	$21,504	$446,974
27	$446,974	$26,818	$23,225	$497,017
28	$497,017	$29,821	$25,083	$551,921
29	$551,921	$33,115	$27,089	$612,125
30	$612,125	$36,728	$29,256	$678,109
31	$678,109	$40,687	$31,597	$750,392
32	$750,392	$45,024	$34,124	$829,540
33	$829,540	$49,772	$36,854	$916,167
34	$916,167	$54,970	$39,803	$1,010,940
35	$1,010,940	$60,656	$42,987	$1,114,583

ASSUMPTIONS:

1. Annual per capita cost of health care is $6,280.

2. Annual growth on savings are calculated at 6%.

3. Annual savings from reduced health care costs are deposited into the portfolio on December 31 of each year, and thus do not figure into the growth of the portfolio for that year. We do it this way to show the most conservative outcome possible.

4. We assume 8% inflation on the costs of health care. As a result, the amount saved each year by reducing said health care costs will also increase by 8% per year.

(Courtesy of William A. Mertes, Chief Financial Officer, American Financial Advisors.)

increased deductibles and co-payments, and the like. This is an exercise to make the point that if we can reduce the national amount spent on medical care by decreasing the number of sick people in our country, then perhaps we don't have to all be spending an extra 15 percent for everything we purchase to cover the cost of medical care. What could 292 million Americans do with an extra $3,140 in their pockets?

In the interest of anticipating some of the skeptics who think this may be too generous, let's get even more conservative in our estimates. Let's go back to the figures that relate specifically to the lifestyle-related conditions mentioned in chapters one through seven. After all, $25,120 represents ALL of health care, and I want to illustrate how, even on extremely conservative estimates, we can still make a tremendous improvement in our personal wealth and national economy by making improvements in our lifestyles.

Our Personal Health Care Bill calculations revealed that for the seven health care issues mentioned, our family of four is spending $13,818 per year. Again, let's use the conservative estimate that making at least one, if not several, lifestyle habit improvements can reduce our risk of disease by only 50 percent. $13,818 divided by four equals $3,454 per person. Decreasing this number by 50 percent equals $1,727. Using this figure, let's see how much we can save over time.

What this shows us is that in the most conservative of projections for a person who makes enough of a lifestyle

Our Personal Health Care Bill
(based on a family of four)

Heart Disease	*$5,520 / year*	*$460 / month*
Cancer	*$2,876 / year*	*$240 / month*
Diabetes	*$1,808 / year*	*$151 / month*
Chronic Pain	*$1,643 / year*	*$137 / month*
Stress	*$ 780 / year*	*$ 65 / month*
Obesity	*$1,027 / year*	*$ 86 / month*
Drug Reactions	*$ 164 / year*	*$ 14 / month*
Total Bill:	**$13,818 / year**	**$1,152 / month**

*(Calculated by taking the total health care cost of these diseases
and dividing it by the total population.)*

change to reduce their risk by only 50 percent, applied only to the amount that we can reasonably say should be effected by improved lifestyle habits, that person can save over a $500,000 over a 35 year period. Who wouldn't like to make a half a million dollars to stay well? It's also important to remember that this is incremental savings. This should be in addition to your traditional savings for your retirement. And again, I remind you that the half a million dollars is just a bonus to the fact that you will enjoy a life of emotional, physical, and social wealth beyond the financial benefit.

How Staying Healthy Can Make You Rich

Seven Lifestyle Conditions

Per Capita Cost of 7 Lifestyle Conditions Reduced by 50%

Year	Beginning Value	6% Growth	Amount Saved Inflated @ 8%	Ending Value
1	$0	$0	$1,727	$1,727
2	$1,727	$104	$1,865	$3,696
3	$3,696	$222	$2,014	$5,932
4	$5,932	$356	$2,176	$8,463
5	$8,463	$508	$2,350	$11,321
6	$11,321	$679	$2,538	$14,537
7	$14,537	$872	$2,741	$18,150
8	$18,150	$1,089	$2,960	$22,199
9	$22,199	$1,332	$3,197	$26,728
10	$26,728	$1,604	$3,452	$31,783
11	$31,783	$1,907	$3,728	$37,419
12	$37,419	$2,245	$4,027	$43,691
13	$43,691	$2,621	$4,349	$50,661
14	$50,661	$3,040	$4,697	$58,398
15	$58,398	$3,504	$5,073	$66,974
16	$66,974	$4,018	$5,478	$76,471
17	$76,471	$4,588	$5,917	$86,976
18	$86,976	$5,219	$6,390	$98,584
19	$98,584	$5,915	$6,901	$111,400
20	$111,400	$6,684	$7,453	$125,538
21	$125,538	$7,532	$8,049	$141,119
22	$141,119	$8,467	$8,693	$158,280
23	$158,280	$9,497	$9,389	$177,166
24	$177,166	$10,630	$10,140	$197,935
25	$197,935	$11,876	$10,951	$220,763
26	$220,763	$13,246	$11,827	$245,836
27	$245,836	$14,750	$12,774	$273,360
28	$273,360	$16,402	$13,795	$303,556
29	$303,556	$18,213	$14,899	$336,669
30	$336,669	$20,200	$16,091	$372,960
31	$372,960	$22,378	$17,378	$412,716
32	$412,716	$24,763	$18,768	$456,247
33	$456,247	$27,375	$20,270	$503,892
34	$503,892	$30,234	$21,892	$556,017
35	$556,017	$33,361	$23,643	$613,021

ASSUMPTIONS:

1. Annual per capita cost of health care represented by 7 Lifestyle Conditions is $3,454. Reduced by 50%, the result is $1,727 per year.

2. Annual growth on savings are calculated at 6%.

3. Annual savings from reduced health care costs are deposited into the portfolio on December 31 of each year, and thus do not figure into the growth of the portfolio for that year. We do it this way to show the most conservative outcome possible.

4. We assume 8% inflation on the costs of health care. As a result, the amount saved each year by reducing said health care costs will also increase by 8% per year.

(Courtesy of William A. Mertes, Chief Financial Officer, American Financial Advisors.)

SPECIAL SECTION

Perspectives on Wellness

Rich People, Poor Planning
By Paul H. Auslander, CFP

In my 25 years of providing financial planning services to high net worth individuals, celebrities, executives, and business owners, I've discovered the most overlooked aspect of building wealth is building health so you can enjoy the fruits of your labor. At American Financial Advisors, providing financial advice to people seeking to build wealth, I have found over the years that what clients really seek is not just more money—they want more life!

In fact, we have helped pioneer new services including "financial-life plans" that assist our clients in creating a lifestyle of building both wealth and health. One of the services we offer is to include vital information specifically related to people's lifestyles. For example, if one of our clients smokes, we will include the reduced life expectancy for smokers, as well as the cost of care, in their financial-life plan, because it helps people have the facts to make better decisions and better plans. If someone doesn't get the hint to stop smoking, they had better at least be financially prepared to pay for the exorbitant cost of treating the cancer they will likely get as a result.

Another service our clients appreciate is that when we create a financial-life plan for someone, we will include the essential costs for services like health club memberships or routine chiropractic care in their plan. We decided long ago that we want to fully serve our clients by including the costs of sickness and wellness in their plans. These are real costs that most financial advisors don't include as part of their services.

Let me share with you some real examples of clients with whom I've consulted over the years.

Client A came to me a little over two years ago to prepare an emergency financial/estate plan. He had created a company that employed 21,000 people in the high-tech industry. He had just been diagnosed with terminal cancer. He was worth $153 million and willing to spend it all on a cure. He was 47 years old, a heavy smoker, and under tremendous stress. He tried to exercise, but couldn't maintain the schedule of doing so. He died early in 2006, and left four children fatherless. Before he died, he spent over $10 million trying every conceivable remedy. Without his leadership, and because his ego was too big to create a succession plan, his company is near bankruptcy, and his wife and children are in serious financial difficulty.

Entrepreneur B was a creative genius and started an enterprise that eventually grew through franchising, providing him and his family with a net-worth in excess of $500 million. He continued to have a minor role in the company after it was sold to a large, multi-national corporation, and started to dabble in high-risk ventures. He enjoyed over ten years of good times, great wealth, and heavy partying. During one of those wonderful events, he crashed his helicopter, survived, but broke his back in three places.

He went through intensive therapy, but only regained the use of the upper third of his body. His assets were still primarily in the stock of the company that bought him out, and they were suffering during the stock market crash from 2000-2002. He was spending over $5 million a year to keep himself and his family comfortable (by their standards). He came to me at this point, on the recommendation of his CPA firm.

It was too late. The market was crashing, he was overspending and not adequately diversified. He had lost millions on ill-fated ventures and died of a massive heart attack—he was 51 at the time.

Executive C is a woman who rose to the zenith of her profession and was the CEO of one of the top-tier accounting/consulting firms in the country. Due to her position, she was constantly entertaining and attending banquet-style functions. Over a fifteen-year period, she gained over 100 pounds, doubled her cholesterol, and was diagnosed with diabetes. As her health declined, she took more time off and made more foolish decisions, culminating with one that almost destroyed her century-old firm, and soon after this, she was fired. That was three years ago, and she still cannot get a job in her profession. Only now is she recognizing the role that her health played in her corporate downfall.

The ability for people to build wealth is absolutely dependent on their focus and attention on their health. Yes, we certainly recognize that accidents happen and that even proper planning does not guarantee that things will work out perfectly every time; but both building wealth and building health are based on time-tested principles that when properly applied, reduce our risks and help most of us most of the time.

As the CEO of our company I can also tell you that this is not just an individual problem. It is a problem that affects everyone: parents, children, employers, employees, everyone. This is a huge issue for corporate America because of the rising health care and health insurance costs.

Most CEOs find this to be the most contentious point when negotiating with unions for long-term benefits. Even well-run companies, like Starbucks, complain that their employee health care costs are their single largest expense!

In addition, employees in a general malaise who are not necessarily sick, but not necessarily well either, are less productive, more depressed, and more likely to cause injury or mistakes. All of this results in a drag on corporate profitability.

However, I am inspired by the recent trend of companies that understand this and are encouraging employees to "live healthy" by serving better meals in company cafeterias, encouraging wellness care, and allowing wellness services on worksites. They all state that costs are initially higher, but fall dramatically as health improves and productivity increases.

I have dedicated my life to helping people achieve their dreams and live their ideal lifestyle. I have seen too many people over the years misplace their priority on material wealth at the expense of the true riches that life has to offer.

Our company is committed to staying on the cutting edge of providing our clients the very best financial-life services that help everyone seeking an overall greater quality of life. It is true: America needs more people less sick. Americans need to *Discover Wellness*.

Ten Steps to Wealth through Health

1. Stay well and fully fund a Health Savings Account as an additional retirement investment vehicle.

2. Stay well and save the money that you would be paying for pharmaceutical co-payments. The average co-payment is $15-$30 per month, and often people are paying much more. Put that money into your health savings account or IRA or invest it. Over time that money will grow with compound interest. Think about *The Automatic Millionaire* by bestselling author David Bach: this is *The Latte Factor*® for drugs.

3. Get a part-time job exercising for money. Teach an exercise class at a local fitness center. You have to exercise anyway: why not get paid to do it? Many people are able to offset the cost of their nutritional supplements by participating in a network marketing program that is also a part-time business and provides additional residual income. Take the extra money and invest it.

4. Redirect the money you spend on things that are destructive to your health into things that are constructive to your health. A pack of cigarettes costs on average $3.80. A pack-a-day habit costs over $100 per month. Stop smoking and invest the money and stay well. How about investing the money you spend on alcohol? Cable TV? Bar night? If you think about it, you can find $25-$100+ per month that you are presently

spending on destroying your health and instead invest it for your future — while kicking the bad habit!

5. Most employers have an arrangement with a local fitness center. If your employer is willing to subsidize you, take the money that you would spend on a membership and invest it while staying well.

6. Most employers offer wellness programs such as smoking cessation, weight loss, and stress management, and even offer incentives to participate, because it is in both of your best interests for you to stay well. Take advantage of any incentives your employer is offering; take the money you would otherwise spend yourself, and invest it.

7. Stop spending money on unhealthy fast food and prepare fresh wholesome meals at home and bring meals to work. It will be both healthier for you and save you thousands of dollars over time.

8. When you feel better, you will save thousands of dollars on over-the-counter medications that are just masking your symptoms anyway. Stay healthier by not living on unnecessary medications, and invest the money for your future.

9. Think about your performance at work. If you felt better and performed better, could you make more money? Would you have the energy to get a part-time job or turn a hobby into a home-based business that could provide additional income?

10. If you have a pre-existing condition and go to change your health insurance, unless you work for a big company, your condition can cost you thousands of dollars in increased premiums—even if it is only a minor condition. Staying well will prevent you from paying these increased premiums. Invest the savings for your financial future.

Discover Wellness Trends

How will our lives change in the future? There are certain wellness trends in place that we can see coming. If we try to look further into the future, we must use our imaginations. Here's what we know. There is no one who can dispute that the cost of medical care is an issue that all Americans face. Analysts predict that American companies that do not control their medical costs will find they can no longer compete in the global marketplace. The competitive advantage most international companies have is that they often benefit from government-sponsored health care programs: these programs limit a company's exposure to the increasing costs of medical care. This is one of several reasons why we must find solutions to America's health care crisis.

The future will bring changes in who pays for medical care and how much they pay. Due to skyrocketing costs of health care and medical insurance, employers have no choice but to figure out how to reduce their expenses. Sooner or later, most of them will be incorporating wellness programs into their employee benefits packages. That's the good news. The bad news is that those companies who do not implement wellness programs will be forced to control costs later by more difficult measures, such as reducing promised benefits to retirees and continuing to increase deductibles and co-payments while reducing benefits to employees. Alternatively, companies will continue to build the cost of health care into the cost of their products: GM says that $1,500 of every car they sell goes toward the cost of employee health benefits. Another drastic step companies will keep taking to reduce costs is firing full-time employees and rehiring part-timers, to eliminate the cost of employee benefits.

Discover Workplace Wellness

Worksite wellness programs, which include exercise, benefit companies by decreasing health care costs, decreasing occupational injuries, improving employee performance, boosting morale, and decreasing employee turnover and absenteeism. They also help companies improve their image and good-will between employees and management, thereby helping to attract and retain the finest workers.

Although most of the evidence in favor of exercise-based worksite wellness programs comes from larger corporations, there is ample evidence that small companies can enjoy compa-rable benefits as well. Although specific outcomes depend on the nature of the business, the most extensively documented and widely experienced benefits are the reduction of employee health risks and reduced absenteeism. The savings from these reductions are usually significant. Most companies have found that the savings from reduced absenteeism alone more than offsets the cost of a health promotion program.

Many companies have implemented exercise-based workplace wellness programs to actively counteract the detrimental physical effects of job stress, and the results from follow-up studies have been remarkable. Companies such as Coors, Steelcase, DuPont, and Control Data have enjoyed a dramatic improvement in productivity and morale and an equally impressive decrease in employee turnover, health care costs, work-related injury, and absenteeism—the very issues that most companies identified as major employee health concerns. As a matter of fact, it is estimated that the average organization realizes a $3.00-$5.00 return on every dollar they invest on exercise-based wellness programs.

Steelcase, a large furniture maker rated as one of the top 100 places to work by Fortune Magazine, enjoyed a significant drop in the number of job-related injuries—up to 50 percent in one department—after just three months of implementing a 20-minute stretching program to help employees warm up before starting work.

The Staywell program implemented by Control Data Corporation in Minneapolis has saved the company an estimated $1.8 million dollars in reduced absenteeism over a six-year period.

In addition to the physical benefits, exercise has been shown to improve psychological functioning, decrease emotional stress, and to elevate mood. Studies reveal that physically active people are likely to be more emotionally stable, to perform better on tests of cognitive functioning, and to report fewer symptoms of anxiety and depression. Exercise also improves self-confidence and self-esteem and decreases the cardiovascular responses to mental stress.

Let's look further into why employer-sponsored wellness plans are the most effective way to address the health care crisis. First let's start with a dose of reality here: it is not news to anyone that everyone can improve their health by exercising more, watching what they eat, and relaxing. Nobody can really say that they can't afford to do those things, as they don't necessarily require a lot of time or money to accomplish, and yet a high percentage of medical expenses are spent on lifestyle-related issues. Our behavior says that adopting wellness habits is not something that most people are likely to do on their own.

There is no doubt an employer benefits when an employee makes better lifestyle choices. Companies are seriously concerned about their profitability, their ability to compete, and in some cases, their ability to stay in business due to health care costs. They don't want to get rid of their employees, so what options do they have? They can continue to pass on the expenses to the employee through increased deductibles, increased co-payments, and decreased benefits. They can pass on the cost to customers through increased prices. Or they can promote wellness in the workplace and provide incentives to employees to improve their lifestyle choices. The inevitable result will be a decreased need for medical care. This is the ultimate solution.

Recommendations for small businesses that may not have the resources of a large corporation can begin with creating a wellness culture. Employers are leaders of their organization and are responsible for creating the workplace culture. Too often, that culture is to be "connected" 24/7, not leaving time for people to rest, recharge, and rejuvenate themselves. In the end, this leads to lower performance, not better performance. Employers can motivate employees through financial incentives or flexible schedules that encourage people to schedule time to take care of themselves without feeling as if they are not focused on work. Employers can set up relationships with local fitness centers, chiropractors, and other wellness specialists who are willing to create special employee programs that often don't have any cost to the employer.

The corporate wellness industry is in the process of exploding. Many wellness providers are overwhelmed with the demand for these types of programs; and at this point many employers have only just begun implementing very basic programs. It will soon be considered best practices for a company to incorporate a wellness program for all employees and their families to benefit from. It could look something like this:

An employer will offer various incentives to employees who voluntarily participate in a wellness program. Presently, incentives could be $25-$50 for filling out a Health Risk Assessment (HRA) questionnaire or making a call to a wellness coach, or the employer may offer to make contributions to an employee's

Health Savings Account (HSA). Some employers have begun saying that in order to receive health benefits, employees must participate in a wellness program. They are not saying every employee must participate in a wellness program, only those who want to receive health benefits provided by the employer.

Sometimes people forget that health benefits are benefits and, in many cases, not requirements. This may seem pretty aggressive to some people, but think about it: if you are going to bear the cost for someone else's health care, would it be appropriate for that person to make whatever choices he or she wants, while you have to foot the bill for the consequences?

Employers will increasingly host wellness expos onsite. At the expo, employees will receive a wellness start-up kit that may include a variety of tools, including wellness information, a pedometer, vitamin sample packs, a recommended wellness calendar, discount passes for local fitness centers, and coupons for local wellness services, such as chiropractic. At the expo, employees can go through a variety of biometric tests to measure their cholesterol, blood pressure, body mass index, glucose levels, spinal alignment, and more. Employees will receive their results in hopes that if they have any early signs of health concerns, they will take action and make better lifestyle choices to proactively improve their condition—instead of thinking that they are just fine, only to eventually develop a health problem due to neglect. By then, it's a problem that costs a lot of time and money to manage.

Discover Wellness Coaching

Another service that is rapidly becoming commonplace is wellness coaching for employers and employees. Wellness coaching is a service to help inform and inspire you to implement the steps that will get you results. Wellness coaches are highly educated and trained in both health education and coaching methods.

This is different than just having a friend who can give you tips when you need them; this is a resource you access to keep you on track and well-informed. The most popular categories in which coaches help people are weight management, exercise, nutrition, stress management, smoking cessation, and pre- and post-natal care. A coach can help you when you are serious about getting results but lack motivation to learn everything and implement it all without help. Everyone who wants to succeed at something has a coach. Athletes, performing artists, even executives often have a coach to help them bring out their very best. You should, too.

Wellness coaches are extremely valuable because they can be a referral source as well. Many wellness coaches have already researched various wellness services and providers and can recommend them to you, saving you many hours of searching for a provider, and improving chances that you will really like the services you receive.

The future of wellness will be affected by the Internet, which will continue to expand its resources that help make it easier to access information, communicate with wellness providers and doctors, and stay up to date with the latest wellness essentials and wellness solutions. Fitness centers will provide technology allowing your personal trainer to customize a program for you that you will be able to access on your home computer and through kiosks located throughout the fitness center. This will let you and your personal trainer keep you on track. You will be able to see your results anywhere you have Internet access; and one day soon it may be common practice to receive discounts on your health insurance because you are working out, just like you receive a safe driver discount on your auto insurance. Technology will help monitor how much and how well you are doing, and you will be rewarded in many ways for making healthy lifestyle choices.

*Employers can learn more about how to reduce the
skyrocketing cost of health care by visiting
DiscoverWellnessCenter.com*

Consumer-Directed Health Care

Health Savings Accounts (HSAs) are a rapidly growing tool in the growing trend towards "consumer-driven" health care: they typically refer to a type of insurance policy with a high deductible and some form of tax-free account. According to Forrester Research, the number of people with this type of account is expected to grow from 2.7 million to 12 million in two years.

Consumer-directed plans give people the choice of how they want to direct their health care spending. For example, a high deductible health care plan that has a Health Savings

Account feature allows people to choose how they spend the money. When you are spending your own money, you choose the doctor whom you want to see, and you become more sensitive to how much things cost—most people in conventional health plans couldn't really care less about how much a procedure actually costs; they are only concerned about how much their deductible and co-payment are.

In the near future more and more HSAs with high deductible health insurance policies will be purchased directly by the consumer and not through their employers. Best selling author and economist Paul Zane Pilzer, in his book *The New Health Insurance Solution*, observes that these plans are growing in popularity.

He explains that the main reason for this is that some people may qualify to purchase health insurance benefits directly for much less than what they have to pay through their employer-sponsored plan. In some cases, employers have programs that will reimburse employees who buy their own health insurance, which translates into substantial savings.

There is also the benefit of employees having their own policies, which they can keep even if they change employers. In addition, once you have one of these plans, your rates cannot be increased due to your health, which is a major concern for people and often keeps them working "just for the benefits."

One of the best features of an HSA is that you can use pre-tax dollars to pay for services such as chiropractic care, as well as for products and services recommended by your chiropractor. This can translate into savings of up to 40 percent or more off the cost of your care. Just another good reason to work with a wellness professional to help you make good decisions about your health.

Another benefit to Health Savings Accounts is that they can be used as an investment vehicle. If you stay healthy and do not use the money in your HSA, the money is yours to keep. You make pre-tax contributions and accumulate interest on your entire contribution. If you begin at an early enough age you can accumulate hundreds of thousands of dollars for your retirement and never have to pay taxes on it.

Critics of consumer-driven health care tools such as Health Savings Accounts say that the problem with these programs is that consumers are not educated enough to direct their own health care decisions and will therefore not be able to make good decisions on how to manage their health. This is yet another great reason to work with a qualified wellness professional who is educated enough to help you make good healthy choices and also to know when you do or do not require expensive medical attention. In some respects the critics are right about this. People do need to become better educated consumers of health and wellness services; they need to find an all-star team of professionals they can afford and trust to help them stay well and make good decisions.

Want to learn more about HSAs and consumer-directed health care so you can save money on wellness care? Visit DiscoverWellnessCenter.com

America's Wellness Revolution

The future of wellness will be both an "evolution and revolution" according to Steve Case, the founder of America Online. He has recently shifted his focus to a new cause: revolutionizing the health care industry. Steve Case is a true visionary. He resigned as the Chairman of the Board of AOL/Time Warner and is now focusing his attention on his next big venture, which he calls Revolution, an investment company that gives more power to consumers. Most significantly, Case is funding Revolution with $500 million of his own money. Some of that money has been invested in health care, wellness, and resorts. About half of it is invested in companies that allow consumers to choose how to spend their money on health care. People will also be able to take advantage of new developments in technology that will allow them to track providers, services, and expenses, and to access their medical records online. Doctors will be able to improve communications, improve efficiency, and reduce mistakes.

In addition to all of this, Steve Case and Revolution have also launched Lime Media, described as "Lime: Healthy Living with a Twist." Lime Media is a 24-hour cable channel, which provides an outlet for emerging leaders in health care to reach viewers. Lime's 24-hour radio network is also carried by Sirius satellite radio and streamed on the Internet.

The new term for the growing market of people concerned about their health and wellness and the environment is LOHAS, Lifestyles of Health and Sustainability. LOHAS is a $228.9

billion US marketplace for goods and services focused on health, the environment, social justice, personal development, and sustainable living. Consumers attracted to this market have been collectively referred to by researcher Paul Ray as "Cultural Creatives." There is a good chance that if you are reading this book, you are part of this rapidly growing group.

Paul Ray found that Cultural Creatives are educated consumers who make conscientious purchasing and investing decisions based on social and cultural values. Cultural Creatives represent approximately 30 percent of adults in America. Steve Case's Revolution is banking on the fact that this will be a rapidly growing marketplace.

Every social, economic, and political indicator leads to the conclusion that America's health care system needs to be overhauled. With all of the lobbying efforts, money, and cronyism provided by the pharmaceutical industry, and with insurance companies dictating to doctors the treatment they can and cannot provide, the only groups that have any incentive to make a change are employers—who are presently footing most of the bill for the high cost of medical insurance—and people just like you and me.

Getting healthy isn't just a good thing to do for yourself; it's good for the country. America can no longer afford to have so many people sick. It affects everyone, because federal programs that provide medical coverage (e.g., Medicare and Medicaid) to those in need are funded by tax dollars. If the costs continue to increase, the taxes will continue to increase. Who do you think is going to foot the bill for that?

Thank You for Discovering Wellness

Discovering wellness is the most effective way for each of us to improve our own health and wealth while also solving America's health care crisis. This does not mean that people will no longer get sick or that we will eliminate all disease. It is not an anti-medicine agenda. It does not solve every problem associated with health care and health care policy. What it does is address the cause of America's health care crisis by reducing the amount of stress on the system. With millions of people less sick and billions of dollars in savings, think about the possibilities. America could regain its global competitive edge once again and have billions of dollars in surplus to invest in jobs, education, and infrastructure improvements.

Companies will thrive with the increased output and improved quality of work produced by a healthier workforce. Stockholders and our economy will benefit with increased profits, stimulating greater investment in new creative ideas and more jobs.

We will have billions of dollars available to fund research and other more effective complementary forms of health care presently not funded by the traditional medical research establishment. We can continue to afford to invest in technology and ideas that may help in the treatment of diseases.

What else can one say about wellness, except that in the end, the quality of your life is your responsibility? It is that simple. We are each responsible for our own health and well-being; and if you have been to the beach lately and seen the shape and size of people, it is obvious that we are not taking this responsibility seriously enough. It is killing us, literally. It can no longer be an option to be "too busy" or not be able to afford the cost of staying well. Continuing to live on medications without addressing the cause of the problem, living with poor posture, pain, increased weight, decreased strength, and too much stress is the prescription for early death, the ultimate expense.

It is important to mention especially to those of the Baby Boomer generation that your actions have the most profound effect on how our health care industry will evolve. Whatever you do, do not ever feel that it is too late. Don't accept that you are just getting old. Don't buy into the story that you have to live on medications for lifestyle-related diseases when there is so much evidence that you can substantially reduce your risks. Please remember that it's never too late to make better choices for your health.

It is my hope that the end of this book is the beginning of your journey—a journey into a world of wellness and self-improvement. It sounds so silly to say, but the better you are, the better you are. Why wouldn't you want that for yourself?

May this book inspire you to make yourself a top priority, may it provide you knowledge and wisdom about the natural power of life, and may you make a greater contribution to the world because of the gift of life that is yours. Thank you for reading this, and I hope it has shifted you in a way that your life will be RICHER because of what you now know.

References
and Research

Introduction - America's Health Care Crisis

1. Warren E. Sick and Broke. *Washington Post.* February 9, 2005.

2. Himmelstein D, Warren E, Thorne D, Woolhandler S. Illness and Injury as Contributors to Bankruptcy. *Health Affairs* web exclusive February 2, 2005.

3. Smith C, Cowen C, Sensenig A. Catlin A., Health Spending Growth Slows in 2004. *Health Affairs* 25:1 (2006):186-196.

4. California Health Care Foundation. *Health Care Costs 101-2005* March 2, 2005.

5. Borger C. et al. Health Spending Projection Through 2015: Changes on the Horizon. *Health Affairs* web exclusive W61:February 22, 2006.

6. Pear R. US Health Care Spending Reaches All-Time High: 15% of GDP. *New York Times*, January 9, 2004.

7. The Henry J. Kaiser Family Foundation. *Employee Health Benefits: 2005 Annual Survey.* September 14, 2005.

8. Herrick D. Why Employee–Based Health Insurance is Unraveling. National Center for Policy Analysis. November 1, 2005.

9. Fidelity Investments, Press Release, 06 March 2006.

10. Smith C, Cowan C, Sensenig A, and Catlin A. Health Spending Growth Slows in 2004. *Health Affairs* 25:1 (2006):186-196.

11. Borger, C., et al., Health Spending Projections Through 2015: Changes on the Horizon. *Health Affairs* web exclusive W61:February 22, 2006.

12. Starfield B. Is US health really the best in the world? *JAMA*, 2000 Jul 26;284(4):483-5. Starfield B. Deficiencies in US medical care. *JAMA*, 2000 Nov 1;284(17):2184-5.

13. *American Hospital Association News.* February 24, 2003.

14. National Center for Health Statistics. *Health, United States, 2005 With Chartbook on Trends in the Health of Americans.* Hyattsville, Maryland: 2005.

15. Barlett D, and Steele J. Health care and the Free Market. *New York Times.* October 30, 2004.

16. Hook J. 44 Million Americans Lack Health Insurance. *Los Angeles Times.* October 4, 1999.

17. Bernard D, Banthin J. Out-of-Pocket Expenditures on Health Care and Insurance Premiums among the Nonelderly Population, 2003. *Statistical Brief #121* March 2006. Agency for Health care Research and Quality, Rockville, Md. http://www.meps.ahrq.gov/papers/st121/ stat121.pdf

18. *American Hospital Association News*. February 24, 2003.

19. Centers for Disease Control and Prevention. *HIV/AIDS Surveillance Report* 2001;13(No. 2), *HIV/AIDS Surveillance Report 2002;14, HIV/AIDS Surveillance Report* 2003;15 and *HIV/AIDS Surveillance Report* 2004;16.

Chapter One - Cardiovascular Disease

1. American Heart Association Nutrition Committee. Diet and lifestyle recommendations revision 2006: a scientific statement from the American Heart Association Nutrition Committee. *Circulation*. 2006 Jul 4; 114(1): 82-96. Epub Jun 19, 2006.

2. U.S. Department of Health and Human Services. *Preventing Chronic Diseases: Investing Wisely in Health*. April, 2003.

3. Heart Disease and Stroke Statistics—2006 Update: A Report From the American Heart Association Statistics Committee and Stroke Statistics Subcommittee. *Circulation*. 2006; 113:e85-e151.

4. Health Care Financing Review, 2003 Medicare and Medicaid Statistical Supplement. www.cms.hhs.gov/review/supp/2003.

5. Thorpe KE, Florence CS, Howard DH, Joski P. The impact of obesity on rising medical spending. *Health Affairs,* 2004;suppl web exclusives: W4-480-6.

Chapter Two - Cancer

1. American Cancer Society. *Cancer Facts & Figures 2006*. Atlanta, GA: American Cancer Society; 2006.

2. Doll R, Peto R. *The Causes of Cancer*. New York:Oxford Press, 1981.

3. McGinnis JM, Foege WH. Actual causes of death in the United States. *JAMA*. 1993; 270:2207-2212.

4. American Cancer Society: *Cancer Facts and Figures*. Atlanta, Ga. 2003. Harvard Center for Cancer Prevention. *Harvard report on cancer prevention volume 1: causes of human cancer*. Cancer Causes Control. 1996; 7: S55.

5. American Cancer Society. *Cancer Facts & Figures 2006*. Atlanta, Ga. 2006.

6. Chang S, Long SR, et al. Estimating the Cost of Cancer: Results on the Basis of Claims Data Analyses for Cancer Patients Diagnosed With Seven Types of Cancer During 1999 to 2000. *Journal of Clinical Oncology*, Vol. 22, No. 17 (September 1), 2004:3524-3530.

7. 2006 International Agency for Research on Cancer. *IARC Handbooks of Cancer Prevention. Volume 8: Fruits and Vegetables*. Lyon, France. IARC Press; 2003.

8. Harvard Center for Cancer Prevention. *Harvard report on cancer prevention volume 1: causes of human cancer*. Cancer Causes Control. 1996; 7:S55.

9. American Cancer Society. Special Section on Obesity in *Cancer Facts & Figures 2000*. Atlanta: American Cancer Society; 2000.

10. Calle E, Rodriquez C, et al. Overweight, obesity, and mortality from cancer in a prospectively studied cohort of US adults. *NEJM*, 2003; 348:1625-1638.

Chapter Three - Diabetes

1. Centers for Disease Control and Prevention. *National diabetes fact sheet: general information and national estimates on diabetes in the United States, 2005.* Atlanta, GA: U.S. Department of Health and Human Services, Centers for Disease Control and Prevention, 2005.

2. American Diabetes Association. *Diabetes 4-1-1: Facts, Figures, and Statistics at a Glance.*

3. Hogan P, Dall F, Nikolov P. American Diabetes Association. Economic Costs of Diabetes in U.S. in 2002. *Diabetes Care,* March 26, 2003 (3): 917-32.

4. Tuomilento, J. et al. Prevention of Type 2 Diabetes Mellitus by Changes in Lifestyle Among Subjects with Impaired Glucose Tolerance. *NEJM,* Vol. 344, May 3,2001:1343-1350.

Chapter Four - Chronic Pain

1. Jacox A, Carr DB, Payne R, et al. Management of cancer pain. Clinical practice guideline no. 9. In: *AHCPR publication No. 94-0592.* Rockville, MD: Agency for Health Care Policy and Research, U.S. Department of Health and Human Services. Public Health Service 1994.

2. American Pain Society. *Chronic Pain in America: Roadblocks to Relief.* www.ampainsoc.org.

3. Araish, Ballock, Calabro, Derwin, Greenwald, Hascall, Iannotti, Knothe, Lefebure, McDevitt. *Basic Research in Arthritis and Prosthetic Perfor-mance.* Lerner Research Institute September 23, 2005.

4. Srikulmontree T. *Osteoarthritis.* American College of Rheumatology Patient Education Task Force. June, 2006.

5. Arthritis Foundation. *Ankylosing Spondylitis Disease Center Conditions and Treatments.* www.arthritis.org.

6. Sukovich, W. New Surgical Trends in Treating Low Back Pain. *Clinical Front.* Spring 2006 issue.

7. Mayo Foundation for Medical Education and Research. *Reliable Information for a Healthier Life.* April 8, 2005 www.mayoclinic.com.

8. American Academy of Pain Medicine and American Pain Society. The Use of Opioids for the Treatment of Chronic Pain. *Clinical Journal of Pain*, Vol. 13, March, 1997:6-8.

9. Medina JL, Diamond S. Drug Dependency in Patients with Chronic Headache. *Headache*, 1977, Vol. 17:12-14.

10. Nurmikko TJ, Nash TB, Wiles JR. Control of chronic pain. *BMJ.* 1998; 317:1438-1441.

11. Milligan K, Lanteri-Minet M, Borchert K, et al. Evaluation of long-term efficacy and safety of transdermal fentanyl in the treatment of chronic noncancer pain. *J Pain.* 2001; 2:197-204.

12. Canine C. Pain, Profit, and Sweet Relief. *Worth.* March, 1997:79-82, 151-157.

Chapter Five - Stress

1. Merritt R. *Stress Management Significantly Reduces Long-Term Costs of Coronary Artery Disease.* American Psychological Association.

2. Perkins A. Saving money by reducing stress. *Harvard Business Review.* 1994;72(6):12.

3. Oltersdorf C. Use It or Lose It. *The Alcalde* January/February 2002.

4. Blumenthal JA, et al. Stress Management and Exercise Training in Cardiac Patients with Myocardial Ischemia: Effects on Prognosis and Evaluation of Mechanisms. *Arch Internal Med* 1997;157:2213-2223.

Chapter Six - Obesity

1. Finkelstein E, Fiebelkorn I, Wang G. National medical spending attributable to overweight and obesity: how much and who's paying? *Health Affairs,* 2003; 3(1):219-226.

2. Centers for Disease Control and Prevention. *Overweight And Obesity: Home*. May 23, 2006.

3. Hedley A, Odgen C, Johnson C, et al. Prevalence of overweight and obesity among US children, adolescents and adults, 1999-2002. *JAMA.* 2004; 291(23):2847-2850.

4. World Health Oganization. *Obesity Preventing and Managing the Global Epidemic*. Geneva (Switzerland): WHO 1977.

5. Mokdad A, Ford E, Bowman B, et al. Prevalence of obesity, diabetes, and obesity-related health risk factors, 2001. *JAMA.* 2003; 289(1): 76-79.

6. Slavkin H. Obesity, Brain and Gonadal Functions, and Osteoporosis. *JADA* 2000;131(5):673-677 2000.

7. Centers for Disease Control and Prevention (CDC) *National Diabetes Fact Sheet.*

8. Berger L. The 10 Percent Solution: Losing a Little Brings Big Gains. *New York Times* June 22, 2003.

9. CDC. *Overweight and Obesity: Economic Consequences.* March 22, 2006.

10. Understanding Adult Obesity. *NIH Publication No. 01-3680.* National Institutes of Health. USDHHS. 2006.

11. CDC Press Room. *Quick Facts Economic and Health Burden of Chronic Disease.* June 16, 2006.

12. National Center for Chronic Disease Prevention and Health Promotion *Preventing Obesity and Chronic Diseases Through Good Nutrition and Physical Activity.* Revised August 2003. www.cdc.gov.

Chapter Seven - Drug Reactions

1. Lazarou J, Pomeranz BH, Corey PN. Incidence of adverse drug reactions in hospitalized patients: a meta-analysis of prospective studies. *JAMA.* 1998 Apr 15; 279(15):1200-5.

2. Ditto AM. Drug allergy. In: Grammer LC, Greenberger PA, eds. *Patterson's Allergic diseases.* 6th ed. Philadelphia: Lippincott Williams & Wilkins, 2002:295.

3. Jick H. Adverse drug reactions: the magnitude of the problem. *J Allergy Clin Immunol* 1984; 74:555-7.

4. Lazarou J, Pomeranz BH, Corey PN. Incidence of adverse drug reactions in hospitalized patients: a meta-analysis of prospective studies. *JAMA* 1998; 279:1200-5.

5. Einarson TR. Drug-related hospital admissions. *Ann Pharmacother* 1993; 27:832-40.

6. Vogt D. Specialist in Social Legislation Domestic Social Policy Division *CRS Report for Congress Direct–To–Consumer Advertising of Prescription Drugs.* March 25, 2005.

7. Vastag B. Pay attention: Ritalin acts much like cocaine. *JAMA*. 2001 Aug 22-29; 286(8): 905-6.

8. Rosenthal MB, Berndt ER, Donohue JM, Frank RG, Epstein AM. Promotion of prescription drugs to consumers. *NEJM*. 2002 Feb 14; 346(7): 498-505.

9. Wolfe SM. Direct-to-consumer advertising—education or emotion promotion? *NEJM*. 2002 Feb 14;346(7):524-6.

10. Mekay E. *What 800 Million Buys on Capitol Hill*. Inter Press Service July 8, 2005.

11. Wolfe SM. Direct-to-consumer advertising—education or emotion promotion? *NEJM*. 2002 Feb 14; 346(7): 524-6.

12. Rabin R. Caution about overuse of antibiotics. *Newsday*. September 18, 2003.

13. For calculations detail, see "Unnecessary Surgery." Sources: HCUPnet, Health care Cost and Utilization Project. Agency for Health care Research and Quality, Rockville, MD. Available at: http://www.ahrq.gov/data/hcup/hcupnet.htm.

14. Manning WG, et al. Inappropriate use of hospitals in a randomized trial of health insurance plans. *N Engl J Med*. 1986 Nov 13;315(20):1259-66. Siu AL, Manning WG, Benjamin B. Patient, provider and hospital characteristics associated with inappropriate hospitalization. *Am J Public Health*. 1990 Oct;80(10):1253-6.

15. US General Accounting Office. Report to the Chairman, Subcommittee on Human Resources and Intergovernmental Relations, Committee on Government Operations, House of Representatives: *FDA Drug Review Postapproval Risks 1976-85*. Washington, DC: US General Accounting Office; 1990:3.

16. Drug giant accused of false claims. *MSNBC News*. July 11, 2003.

17. Ismail MA. Drug Lobby Second to None: How the pharmaceutical industry gets its way in Washington. *The Center for Public Integrity.* July 7, 2005.

18. Ernst FR, Grizzle AJ. Drug-related morbidity and mortality: updating the cost-of-illness model. *J Am Pharm Assoc*. 2001 Mar-Apr;41(2):192-9.

19. Wolfe SM, Sasich LD, Lurie P. *Worst Pills Best Pills: A Consumers Guide to Avoiding Drug-Induced Death or Illness*. 3 ed., 1999. Simon & Schuster: New York.

Chapter Nine - Alignment

1. *Chiropractic Patient Satisfaction and Utilization: A Review of the Current Research*. Foundation for Chiropractic Education and Research Publication #9677, June, 1996.

2. Manga P, Angus D, Papadopoulos C, Swan W. *The effectiveness and cost-effectiveness of chiropractic management of low-back pain*. Ottawa, Ontario, Canada: Pran Manga & Associates, Inc., University of Ottawa, 1993; 65-70.

3. Bigos S, Bowyer O, Braen G, et al. *Acute low back pain in adults. Clinical practice guideline No. 14*. AHCPR Publication No. 95-0642. Rockville, MD: Agency for Health Care Policy and Research, Public Health Service, U.S. Department of Health and Human Services. December, 1994.

4. Coulter ID, Adams AH. Consensus Methods, Clinical Guidelines, and the RAND Study of Chiropractic. *ACA J Chiro*, 1992; 50-61.

5. Shekelle PG. What Role for Chiropractic in Health Care? *NEJM*, 1998; 339(15):1074-1075.

Chapter Sixteen - Staying Healthy Can Make You Rich!

1. Kaiser Public Opinion Spotlight. December, 2005. http://www.kff. org/spotlight/healthcosts/index.cfm.

2. Smith C, Cowan C, Sensenig A, and Catlin A. Health Spending Growth Slows in 2004. *Health Affairs* 2006; 25(1):186-196.

3. Clark K. The Case for Healthcare: AOL founder Steve Case says he wants a revolution—in healthcare. *US News & World Report.* October 17, 2005.

A Note on Personal Cost Calculations for Each Disease:

The "Personal Health Care Bill" amount for each disease was calculated by taking the most current reported total cost of a particular disease and dividing it by 292 million—the estimated total US Population as of January, 2006, according to the US Census.

The source of the total cost of each disease is listed below and can be found listed in this section of references:

	Total cost	**Source**
Heart Disease	*$403 billion*	*Health Affairs 25:1, 2006*
Cancer	*$210 billion*	*Cancer Facts & Figures 2006*
Diabetes	*$132 billion*	*Diabetes Care, March 26, 2003*
Chronic Pain	*$120 billion*	*Clinical Journal of Pain, v.13, 1997*
Stress	*$57 billion*	*Harvard Business Review. v.72, 1994*
Obesity	*$75 billion*	*Centers for Disease Control, 2006*
Drug Reactions	*$12 billion*	*JAMA, v.279, 1998*

Help Yourself by Helping Others Discover Wellness

Discover Wellness, How Staying Healthy Can Make You Rich is the ideal tool to introduce your employees to the benefits of creating better health through better living. Informative and inspirational, *Discover Wellness* is a gift you can give as a health care benefit that benefits you both. Give your employees the incentive they need to do the right thing.

• *Special pricing available for quantities of 10 or more!* •

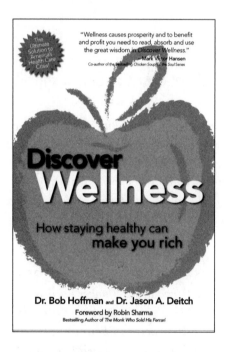

To order additional copies of the Discover Wellness book, please call
The Masters Circle at 1.800.451.4514

Personalize Your Own Discover Wellness Book

A great way to help improve the health of your organization is to personalize your own version of the *Discover Wellness* book. You can add your personalized message as a preface to the book and even place your organization's information in the back of the book.

For details on how you can personalize copies of Discover Wellness with your organization's unique message, please contact Center Path Publishing at 1.952.220.2633

Discover Wellness Book Clubs

Nationwide, wellness doctors, wellness specialists and people of all ages have been creating local *Discover Wellness* book clubs to make getting well a social event. The power of getting well with a group of people is beyond measure. Not only does it make adopting healthy habits much more fun than trying to do it alone, it guarantees your success. The secret to successfully creating better health through better living is not in knowing what to do, it is in being accountable to someone besides yourself.

Contact us by visiting DiscoverWellnessCenter.com if you would like to find or start a *Discover Wellness* book club in your community, organization or workplace. We can even offer you a wellness doctor or professional to guide your club towards success.

Discover Wellness Today

Receive the latest tools, technology and techniques to staying healthy and getting rich. Stay connected, informed and inspired to live your best life with effective strategies and powerful tools to help make your wellness journey a successful adventure.

Subscribe to Discover Wellness Today at DiscoverWellnessCenter.com

Keynote Speeches and Wellness Workshops

Dr. Bob Hoffman, Dr. Jason A. Deitch and their team of wellness doctors and professionals are available for your seminars and meetings. Presentations are rich with information, inspiration and practical tips to immediately begin experiencing the benefits of a wellness lifestyle.

Contact us at DiscoverWellnessCenter.com or 1.800.451.4514 to schedule a speaker who can inspire your crowd to stay healthy and get rich.

Chief Wellness Officer

Stop the bleeding and start the healing of your business' profitability. You don't have to suffer the chronic stress of skyrocketing health care costs anymore. Dr. Bob Hoffman, Dr. Jason A. Deitch and our team of trained wellness doctors and benefits consultants can prescribe exactly what your company needs to get better, faster.

We provide a selection of services that put the "health" back into health care benefits. Our wellness programs are cost-effective, easy to deploy and custom-designed to help you reach your organization's specific goals. You will experience relief, when we help you customize a unique wellness program for your company that will improve morale, increase performance, and make you money. Programs are available for groups of five to 500,000+ in all industries.

Visit DiscoverWellnessCenter.com or call 1.800.451.4514 ext. 157 and request to speak with the Chief Wellness Officer.

Resources for Human Resource Executives

Are you seeking best-in-class wellness products and programs for your employees or employers? We can help you. Our onsite, online and telephonic wellness coaching and concierge services can help you stay informed about the latest tools, technologies, and techniques that can help you help others to take control of their health care costs, increase productivity, and maximize profits.

Discover how you can provide cost-effective, results-driven solutions to your employees or clients today. Visit DiscoverWellnessCenter.com "Corporate Wellness/Small Business Solutions" or call 1.800.451.4514 ext. 157 and request to speak with the Chief Wellness Officer.

Resources for Wellness Professionals

Wellness professionals seeking to grow their practice and enrich their lives will benefit from the experience of the world's largest leadership, training, and practice building firm for chiropractic wellness doctors and wellness professionals in all disciplines. Based on the premise that "success comes from you, not to you" and that "who you are determines how well what you do works" our unique identity-based coaching program will help you make your personal and professional dreams come true.

Visit DiscoverWellnessCenter.com "For Professionals Only" section or call us today at The Masters Circle 1.800.451.4514 and ask for Dr. Robert Kleinwaks to discover more.

Resources for the Wellness Industry

Do you have a business in the wellness industry that you are looking to take to the next level? Discover how we can help you become an industry leader. Our consulting services and networking opportunities help accelerate your wellness company's growth and success. Contact us to find out if your business would benefit from being a part of our network of best-in-class wellness products and services.

Visit DiscoverWellnessCenter.com or call 1.800.451.4514 ext. 157 and request to speak with the Chief Wellness Officer.

Visit the Discover Wellness Blog

Visit our blog at DiscoverWellnessCenter.com to share how *Discover Wellness* has positively impacted your life. Join thousands of other readers all seeking to be well and wealthy. Let us know how much better it feels to be in more control of your health and your health care dollars. Share with us how much weight you have lost and how much self-confidence you have found. We want to hear how your relationships have improved, how your life is better and of course, please share with us the new ways you are discovering how staying healthy is making you rich.